F

HEINEMANN MEDICAL

STUDENT REVIEWS

PRIMARY CARE

D1799795

F003924

Series Editor: Professor Peter Richards MA, MD, PhD, FRCP
Professor of Medicine and Dean, St Mary's Hospital
Medical School, University of London

!

Heinemann Medical
Student Reviews

Primary
Care

Edited by
BRIAN JARMAN
PhD, FRCP, FRCGP
Professor of Primary Health Care, St Mary's Hospital
Medical School, University of London

Heinemann Professional Publishing

Heinemann Medical Books
An imprint of Heinemann Professional Publishing Ltd
Halley Court, Jordan Hill, Oxford OX2 8EJ

OXFORD   LONDON   MELBOURNE   AUCKLAND

First published 1988

© Brian Jarman 1988
British Library Cataloguing in Publication Data
Primary care.—(Heinemann medical student
  reviews).
  1.   General practice
  I.   Jarman, Brian
  362.1′72
  ISBN 0–433–00028–7

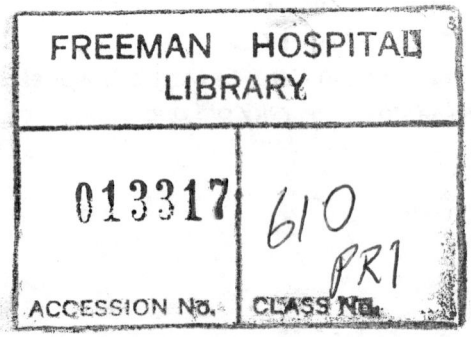
Typeset by Wilmaset, Birkenhead, Wirral and
printed in Great Britain by Biddles Ltd, Guildford

Contents

Contributors

Ms Sarah Castle   Research Assistant
St Mary's Hospital Medical School
University of London
Lisson Grove Health Centre
LONDON NW8 8EG

Professor Andrew Haines   Department of Primary Health Care
University College and Middlesex School of
    Medicine
Highgate Wing
Whittington Hospital
Highgate Hill
LONDON N19 5HT

Dr John Horder   Past President of Royal College of General
    Practitioners
Visiting Professor
Royal Free Hospital School of Medicine
LONDON NW3 2PF

Professor Brian Jarman   Professor of Primary Health Care
St Mary's Hospital Medical School
University of London
Lisson Grove Health Centre
LONDON NW8 8EG

Professor D J Pereira Gray   Professor of General Practice
Postgraduate Medical School
University of Exeter
Barrak Road
EXETER

Dr Patrick Pietroni   Senior Lecturer
St Mary's Hospital Medical School
University of London
Lisson Grove Health Centre
LONDON NW8 8EG

Ms Jennie Popay   Senior Lecturer
Thomas Coram Research Unit
University of London Institute of Education
41 Brunswick Square
LONDON WC1N 1AZ

Preface

The term 'primary health care' is not one which is immediately understood by the general public or used much in everyday speech. In the UK people use the terms 'general practitioner', 'family doctor' or just 'my doctor' when talking about doctors who look after people in the community and the terms 'district nurse' or 'health visitor' for community nurses. So, for practical purposes, in the UK, primary health care can be thought of as care provided by general practitioners, who are part of the Family Practitioner Services, and by the community health services of health authorities, particularly health visitors, district nurses and domiciliary midwives, physiotherapists, occupational and speech therapists, and chiropody services. However, hospital accident and emergency departments, child health and school health services, local authority social services and the other Family Practitioner Services (dental, pharmaceutical and ophthalmic) also have an important role to play and are often the first point of contact for primary care.

The WHO definition of primary health care is 'essential health care based on practical, scientifically sound and socially acceptable methods and technology, made universally available to individuals and families in the community through their full participation and at a cost that the community and the country can afford to maintain at every stage of their development in the spirit of self-reliance and self-determination'. In developing countries, where doctors and trained nurses are often few and far between, village health workers, nursing aids, health promoters, barefoot doctors and others with varying degrees of medical and nursing training provide much of the primary care which is available in the community. They often have an emphasis on preventive services and are far removed from the hospitals which concentrate on treatment services. These topics are discussed in the chapter on primary care in developing countries.

The first chapter of this book traces the evolution of the general practitioner services in the UK over the last two centuries. This has led to the development of a unique system of personal doctors providing universal coverage for virtually the whole of the population, free at the time that it is given, with a very even geographical distribution throughout the community. It is a system which integrates preventive and treatment services and is provided at a relatively low cost, paid for mainly from taxation. In fact it fulfils most of the WHO criteria for good primary care services but in addition adds the advantages of a personal doctor giving continuing care over many years to individuals and their families. It should not be forgotten however that this has not occurred by chance but as a result of many years of negotiating and bargaining between the Government and representatives of the profession such as the BMA, the RCGP (and at the time of the Family Doctors' Charter in 1965, the Medical Practitioners' Union) and by consultation processes which have allowed members of the public to have some say, for instance in the debates which led up to the 1987 White Paper on improving primary health care. This White Paper is discussed, in particular the way in which it tackles the problems of setting standards, community involvement, patient participation and increasing health promotion. The complex problems of inner cities are dealt with in a separate chapter.

Other chapters cover undergraduate and postgraduate medical education, the primary care team and prescribing, epidemiology and prevention in general practice. Consultation skills and the doctor–patient relationship are important aspects of the way general practitioners work and are covered in a separate chapter. This leads on to a chapter on self care and here other forms of primary care and the holistic approach are brought in.

In this book we have tried to take a broad look at primary care and, rather than concentrating in detail on individual diseases and their management, to consider also how social factors are related to problems which are encountered in the primary care setting. The introduction of social factors extends the scope of the book beyond primary *health* care to other forms of primary care and social medicine and so we have used the title Primary Care for the book.

I would like to express my gratitude to Professor Brian Abel Smith, Dr John Ball, Dr John Oldroyd and Dr Michael Wilson for reading the chapter on the development of general practice and to Professor Andrew Herxheimer and various people in the prescribing division of the DHSS for reading the chapter on prescribing. Nicola Dollimore and Dr Paul Wallace kindly read the whole manuscript in the draft stage. All of these people have made valuable suggestions, but I and the contributors to individual chapters of course bear the responsibility for any errors or omissions and for the opinions expressed. Finally I would like to thank the members of the St Mary's Department of General Practice and members of my own practice working in Lisson Grove Health Centre and to my wife and family for all the help and support that they have provided.

Brian Jarman, 1988

Chapter

1

The Development of General Practice in the UK

HISTORICAL DEVELOPMENT • BASIC PRINCIPLES OF GENERAL PRACTICE IN THE UK TODAY

'The essential unit of medical practice is the occasion when in the intimacy of the consulting room or sick room, a person who is ill, or believes himself to be ill, seeks the advice of a doctor whom he trusts.' Sir James Spence.

The evolution of general practice as we know it in the UK today, in which everyone has their own personal doctor, was a long, and at times painful, process. The key developments were the *National Health Insurance Act* of 1911, the *National Health Service* which started in 1948 and the *Family Doctor Charter* of 1966. The Government's White Paper on improving primary health care published in 1987 promises also to be influential.

HISTORICAL DEVELOPMENT

With the dissolution of the monasteries at the Reformation in the sixteenth century there was a change of medical care provision from the Church, which had previously provided services in monasteries and priories, to the State. The *Royal College of Physicians* was founded in 1518 and the *United Barber-Surgeons' Company* in 1540. The *Royal College of Surgeons* received its Royal Charter in 1800. The doctors who worked in the hospitals became Members and Fellows of the Royal Colleges of Medicine and Surgery, whereas the group of practitioners who practised outside hospital were originally the apothecaries and were eventually to become known in the UK as general practitioners. The *Society of Apothecaries* received its Royal Charter in 1617 and the Apothecaries Hall, which was originally built by Dominican monks in 1276, was bought by the Apothecaries Society in 1632. It was destroyed in the Great Fire of London and rebuilt in 1688, and the building exists today almost unchanged.

In Europe, similar divisions developed between the doctors who became specialists or consultants and did at least part of their work in hospitals, and those who practised in the community. In Britain, specialists generally did their hospital work on a voluntary basis and received their income from private consultations for which they were able to charge considerably higher fees than the general practitioners. Gradually, it came to be accepted as medical etiquette for specialists to see only those cases which were referred to them by general practitioners. The wealthy received specialist advice from physicians and surgeons and the poor were able to obtain specialist attention in voluntary hospital outpatient departments. The apothecaries, who had developed from grocers, originally received their income from dispensing drugs and, until 1829, they were not allowed to charge for the medical advice which they gave (rather like the pharmacists today).

The 1858 *Medical Act* enabled all doctors – physicians, surgeons, general practitioners and apothecaries – to have their names placed on the *Medical Register*, which allowed members of the public to identify qualified medical practitioners. With the development of scientific medicine in the nineteenth and twentieth centuries, the role of the specialist became increasingly important. The class divisions within the profession were perpetuated because only those who could afford the long periods of low paid hospital apprenticeships could afford to become specialists, while the less well-off students became general practitioners.

Club practice

The system of general practice care based on the panel system, which was started with the 1911 National Health Insurance (NHI) Act of Lloyd George, was adopted in a modified form nationally at the beginning of the National Health Service (NHS) in 1948. However, before the NHI Act there had been a system of *club practice* which was started by friendly societies.

The friendly societies developed from the beginning of the nineteenth century. They were clubs of working men who met for social reasons, but they also provided their members with a form of insurance against sickness and hired doctors to certify incapacity for work. These club doctors were paid by capitation according to the number of members in the club, and they gave general medical care as well as sickness certificates to the club members. In the tradition of the apothecaries they also dispensed medicines. Club doctors could also take private patients and younger general practitioners would depend on their club practice until they could build up a list of private patients, rather in the same way that specialists depended on honorary appointments in the voluntary hospitals while they were building up their private practice.

Club practice gradually spread throughout the country until about one third of the working population was covered (dependants were usually excluded) and roughly half the general practitioners were engaged in this type of practice, a quarter of them receiving most of their income by this means. For a fee of two to four shillings (£0.10 to £0.20 – there was only a small increase throughout the nineteenth century), the club doctor provided general medical services and drugs for a year. If members of the club were dissatisfied with the doctor he was dismissed, and doctors had little say in the running of the friendly societies. Specialists supported the club system because it limited the number of general practitioners who were tempted to specialize, particularly as the referral system developed.

National Health Insurance Act 1911

By 1911 it had become clear to some of the club doctors in the British Medical Association that, in order to break the stronghold which the friendly societies had over them, it would be necessary for them to accept the Lloyd George National Health Insurance Act which aimed to introduce a state system of panel doctors. Under this system each doctor was able to build up a *panel list* of patients of any size he desired (limits were imposed in 1920) once he had been accepted by the local administration (called the insurance committee). Doctors continued to be paid by capitation fee, although this was increased from four shillings to seven shillings, but they ceased to be responsible for the dispensing of drugs and merely needed to write prescriptions which, in most cases, were dispensed by chemists. Patients had free choice of general practitioners and similarly the doctors were able to refuse to accept patients onto their list. Doctors had considerable freedom in the type of services that they provided and could not be dismissed without the right to an extensive appeal procedure.

The NHI Act covered all manual workers plus non-manual workers whose income was below a certain limit (£160 in 1911, increasing to £420 in 1942). Those eligible over the age of 16 years (and from 1937 over the age of 14 years) could be covered in return for the payment of weekly contributions which were automatically deducted from their wages (as National Insurance deductions are made these days). The workers paid four pence (4d, about £0.02) per week and their employers and the state contributed five pence per week, enabling the employee to get what Lloyd George called 'nine pence for four pence'. These weekly insurance contributions covered most of the costs of the system. As a result of later extensions to include the unemployed and other groups, the number of people covered by the NHI Act rose from one third of the population in 1913 to one half of the population in 1942. Dependants of the manual workers and those non-manual workers with an income above the threshold limit were not covered by the Act. The benefits provided for those who were insured were sickness benefit – ten shillings (£0.50) a week for men and seven shillings and sixpence (£0.375) a week for women for the first twenty-six weeks of illness, after which it became disablement benefit at five shillings per week – and maternity benefit of thirty shillings on the birth of a child. For medical treatment, the insured panel patients received general medical care from general practitioners and medicines without charge for life (the cash benefits stopped at the age of 70 years in 1911 and at the age of 65 years in 1925).

Thus, the NHI Act provided for general practitioner treatment for insured persons, but hospital and specialist treatment was excluded (except for tuberculosis treatment in a sanatorium). The dependants of the insured persons had to pay for their treatment or be treated as a charity case in a voluntary hospital, or alternatively they received general practitioner care under the auspices of the *Poor Law* (after passing a strict means test) from general practitioners who also practised part-time as district medical officers. In order to provide medical cover for the dependants of people covered by the NHI Act, local authorities began to provide free services, such as maternity and child care, and isolation hospitals. This provision gradually increased the proportion of the population covered by free medical care.

A salaried service and the Dawson Report

The *Ministry of Health* was started by Lloyd George in 1919. This unified the state medical provision under the Poor Law, the local authorities and the panel system into one government department. With the formation of a Ministry of Health, there was pressure from unions for the introduction of a salaried general practitioner service because they considered that doctors were becoming too dependent on the insurers and employers, and they believed that by removing this influence the workers would receive fairer assessment of their accident compensation claims. It was felt that if the doctors were paid by means of a state medical service then they would be less under the influence of employers and insurance companies. The friendly societies also saw that a state medical service would be one way of providing medical cover for the dependants of the people covered by insurance. Women, who were increasingly more vocal at this time of the fight for female suffrage, were also in favour of a state salaried service as they were the ones who were most likely to be excluded from the provisions of the NHI Act. Doctors were, on the whole, unsympathetic to the salaried system, partly because they felt that many of the medical clubs run by workers had been particularly harsh on doctors and had been unsympathetic to their requests for increased income for doctors. In 1918 a consultant physician, Sir Bertrand (later Lord) Dawson, suggested that the insurance system should be adapted to cover a wider section of the community and thus avoid the threat of the introduction of a state salaried system. Some salaried posts, mainly for preventive work, were to be allowed in local authority clinics but the main aim was to extend the NHI panel system.

Lord Dawson also produced a report, the *Dawson Report*, which came out in 1920 and was based on the idea of doctors working in teams from a network of well equipped health centres. It was planned that the health centres should contain a general practice with consulting rooms and diagnostic X-ray and laboratory facilities, and also local authority clinics and a number of beds for patients. The larger health centres were to contain more elaborate diagnostic facilities and would provide facilities for consultations by specialists. However, the organization of medical care suggested in the Dawson Report was not implemented at that time, partly because of the fear of the doctors that the extension of free medical care and greater state control would eventually lead to a salaried service. Another factor was the financial situation in 1920 which made it difficult to increase expenditure on social reforms that the country could not afford, the provision of hospital beds suggested in the Dawson Report being a particularly expensive element. It was not until the Family Doctors' Charter of 1966 that the health centre idea started to take shape in any significant way, and then it was without the inclusion of beds.

As an extension of the negotiations on the Dawson Report before the formation of the NHS in the early 1940s, there was a suggestion that the health centres should be run by general practitioners employed entirely on a salaried basis by local authorities. This suggestion was also strongly opposed by general practitioners who were wary of being employees of local authorities.

The Beveridge Report and the National Health Service 1948

In the tough negotiations which led to the formation of the National Health Service, the first suggestion was that of an extension of free general practitioner care to the dependants of insured persons and the principle of group practice in health centres, with the general practitioners who worked there being paid partly by a salary and partly by capitation. General practitioners were to be paid pensions and the sale of practices would be abolished. The health centres would also offer specialist consultations and the normal range of services from local authority clinics. It was planned that the National Health Service should be free and open to all.

The general practitioners were not in favour of local authority control of the health centres; they wished to have a national system with administrative control at the local level in which they were themselves involved. It was eventually agreed that the administration of general practitioner services would continue using a method similar to that employed under the NHI Act involving a panel system of insurance committees with their local medical committees. Having obtained government agreement to this form of administration, the doctors agreed to the introduction of a National Health Service providing universal coverage.

Apart from introducing universal coverage, abolishing the sale of practices and introducing controls over the distribution of general practitioners, the panel system of general practice continued almost unchanged after the introduction of the NHS in 1948. Even though Aneurin Bevan considered the family doctor to be the most important part of the health service, he did not provide for methods of improving standards in general practice. Doctors and other professionals formed about 50% of the membership of the *Executive Councils* (called *Family Practitioner Committees* after the 1974 NHS reorganization) which administered general practitioner affairs. The general practitioners on this committee were from the *Local Medical Committee* – an elected group of doctors in each area meeting regularly to discuss professional matters. There was also a subcommittee of the executive council to consider complaints from patients which ensured a fair hearing for both patients and doctors. NHS doctors were allowed to do private practice – although this did not affect general practice a great deal as most people chose to be treated under the NHS. The payment to general practitioners was entirely by capitation without the additional salary element which Bevan had wished to introduce.

The Family Doctor Charter 1966 and beyond

The period from the beginnings of the NHS in 1948 to the time of the so called Family Doctors' Charter of 1966, was one of relative decline for general practice and relative rise for the increasingly technical and scientific hospital services. The proportion of gross NHS expenditure devoted to *General Medical Services* (general practitioner services) dropped from 10.1% in 1949 to 7.5% in 1966. The capitation system of payment meant that there was strong competition between general practitioners for patients but no incentive, once a patient was on the list, to provide good services – in fact the reverse was the case, in that the more services the doctor provided the less was his net income likely to be.

In 1965, general practitioners forced the Government (by threatening to resign *en masse* from the NHS) to make a considerable number of improvements which transformed the general practitioner service to the way it is today. The basic panel system was retained but the capitation element of a general practitioner's pay was reduced to about 50% and a form of salary equivalent (known as a *Basic Practice Allowance*) was introduced. There were also payments for practising in groups of three or more doctors, and reimbursements for the costs of premises and for 70% of the costs of employing up to two members of ancillary staff per general practitioner for receptionist, secretarial and nursing work. There were payments for immunizations and cervical smears but these only formed a small proportion of a doctor's pay. It was agreed that the career earnings of a doctor entering into general practice would be about the same as those of a doctor who chose to become a specialist. *The Royal College of General Practitioners* (which had been formed in 1952 and received its Royal Charter in 1972) and the General Medical Services Committee of the BMA pushed for a three-year period of required vocational training (two years in approved hospital jobs and one year in an approved training practice) which was formally introduced in 1981–2.

As a result of this long period of evolution there exists in the UK a system of general practice in which virtually the whole population is registered with a general practitioner of their choice and services are free at the time they are received. The ideals expressed by Sir James Spence are available to the whole population.

BASIC PRINCIPLES OF GENERAL PRACTICE IN THE UK TODAY

Most of the arrangements for the provision of general practitioner services in the UK are laid down in the *1974 Statutory Instrument NHS (General Medical and Pharmaceutical Services) Regulations* and in the *Statement of Fees and Allowances for General Practitioners* (the Red Book). This is constantly being updated as a result, usually, of changes which arise from debates at the Annual Conference of Local Medical Committees and from negotiations between the Government and the General Medical Services Committee of the *British Medical Association*. The key features of the system are:

(1) Patients *register* with their own personal general practitioner. A patient can register with only one general practitioner at a time but has free choice of the general practitioners in the area and can change doctors at any time. The patient effects registration by handing their medical record card to the new general practitioner: the signing of this card by the patient and doctor forms a contract for the doctor to provide general medical services for that patient. The card is sent by the doctor to the local Family Practitioner Committee and this is the mechanism by which payment to the new doctor is initiated and payment to the previous doctor is stopped and the medical records are transferred from the previous doctor to the new doctor. The general practitioner has the right not to accept a patient and may also remove a patient from the list. A mechanism exists for allocating

patients to general practitioners if they have difficulty being accepted onto a list. Lists of general practitioners are available in public libraries, post offices and elsewhere.

(2)   The doctor receives a *fixed payment,* or Basic Practice Allowance, plus a *capitation fee* per person registered (with increments for patients aged 65–74 years and for those aged 75 years or more). On average, the capitation fees constitute about 50% of a doctor's income, the Basic Practice Allowance (which is reduced pro rata if the doctor has less than 1000 patients on the list) forms about 25%, and payments for practising in a group, for immunization and cervical smears etc. form the remainder. The NHS also provides a superannuation scheme to provide general practitioners with an NHS pension (see pp. 86–7).

(3)   The general practitioner is *reimbursed* for the cost of premises (rent and rates up to agreed limits) and for 70% of the cost of members of ancillary staff doing reception, secretarial, clerical and nursing work with the practice patients (also up to agreed limits).

(4)   Arrangements exist to enable general practitioners to build, purchase and improve their own *premises* and this can be financially advantageous for the general practitioner. However, since the mid-1960s an increasing proportion of general practitioners (at present about a quarter) have chosen to work in health centres provided by the local health authority in conjunction with health authority staff – mainly district nurses and health visitors, but also community physiotherapists, chiropodists, dentists, speech therapists and so on.

(5)   The health visitors and district nurses attached to a particular practice work mainly with the patients of that practice as part of the *primary care team.* Since the introduction of neighbourhood nursing based on geographical patches, as the result of a review of community nursing by a committee chaired by Mrs Julia Cumberlege in 1986, there has been a need for clarification about how this nursing arrangement fits in with the primary care team concept. Practice attached nurses work with patients registered with a practice who will live near the practice but not exactly within a clearly defined geographical nursing patch. However, it is possible to allow a degree of flexibility whereby attached nurses are permitted to cross nursing patch boundaries in the majority of cases. For the few patients who live outside the patch and also

have high nursing needs, it is possible to devise reciprocal arrangements with the nurse managers of adjoining patches to deal with these patients' nursing needs.

(6) The general practitioner takes 24 hour, 365 days per year *responsibility* for the general medical care of all the patients registered with him or her. A deputy may be used for medical cover out of normal working hours up to agreed limits, but the arrangements and costs are the responsibility of the general practitioner. There is a payment to general practitioners for this cover out of normal working hours which, in theory, the general practitioner can choose not to accept (and not to provide 24 hour services) if alternative arrangements can be made. In practice, this is usually not possible and the general practitioner is responsible for full-time continuing cover.

(7) General practitioners are responsible for their medical *practice expenses* for cars, home telephones, basic medical equipment and so on. As they are independent practitioners, and therefore considered for tax purposes as self-employed, they can offset these practice expenses against tax. In health centres in particular, more sophisticated equipment, such as that required for some laboratory tests, is often provided by the local health authority.

(8) *Referral* of the patient to a specialist for an opinion or for admission to hospital is done by the general practitioner rather than allowing the patient direct access to hospital. This applies on all occasions except for accidents and emergencies, sexually transmitted diseases and drug addiction.

(9) The *medical notes* of the patient are transferred, in the manner described above, to the new general practitioner when the patient changes doctor so that, in theory, the general practitioner has the patient's lifetime medical history ('cradle to the grave' or 'womb to tomb' notes). The notes should include those made by previous general practitioners as well as hospital discharge summaries and the opinions of specialists to whom the patient has been referred in the past. This should apply to all of a patient's past medical experience because of the rules of medical etiquette whereby a patient is considered to have only one main generalist doctor (their general practitioner) at a time, other doctors seeing the patient only after referral by the general practitioner – or in an emergency, in which case they write later to the patient's general practitioner.

(10) *Medical care is free at the time that it is given* and is paid for from general taxation and by National Insurance contributions from the employer and employee (the principle of shared risks).

(11) Full 24 hour/365 days per year cover by the general practitioner for an average list of NHS patients cannot easily be combined with care for a significant number of private patients. Mixed private and NHS general practice is not allowed, and patients who are registered with a general practitioner under the NHS cannot also be treated by that doctor as a private patient. In the UK, the *General Household Survey* has shown that only about 1% of general practitioner consultations are with private patients (see Table 2.1, p. 18).

(12) The *administration* of medical records, doctors' pay, discipline and standards of service, appointment of new doctors, allocation of patients, supervising deputizing services and so on, is dealt with by the Family Practitioner Committee, which is serviced by administrators who are employees of the NHS. The committee is made up of members of the general public, the professions (mainly general practitioners) and representatives of the NHS.

(13) The capitation system can lead to competition between doctors to attract patients onto their lists. This may not ensure that the quality of the service provided is up to scratch, but there are some methods of *quality control* which include:

- inspection of premises to ensure that they are up to standard for reimbursement for rent and rates
- inspection of medical records and practices for training practices
- monitoring of the availability of general practitioners from the surgery hours published in the medical list (these must be spread evenly throughout the week and the general practitioner must be available for a minimum number of hours per week to see patients)
- a patient complaints system whereby written complaints must be investigated if they are made within a reasonable time (in practice about three months)
- the existence of the *Community Health Council* in each district to which patients with problems regarding general practitioner and other health services can go for advice and help
- for patients choosing a doctor, the Medical Register – pub-

lished annually and available in public libraries – lists doctors'
training, qualifications, publications and so on.

(14) There are arrangements for obtaining an equitable *distribution
of doctors* throughout the country. The *Medical Practices Committee*, formed at the time of the NHS in 1948, controls the
distribution of general practitioners by monitoring the average
size of doctors' lists over small areas, of average population
about 40 000 people, throughout the country. At the present
time, the average general practitioner is responsible for about
2000 patients. In areas where the average list size (corrected for
'inflation' of lists) is below 1700 patients, known as 'restricted'
areas, no new doctors are allowed to practise in the NHS. For
list sizes between 1700 and 2100, 'intermediate' areas, new
doctors wishing to practice in the area must put up a case
before the Medical Practices Committee to justify the need for
their services. Where the average list size is between 2100 and
2500, 'open' areas, doctors are free to practise without restriction by the Medical Practices Committee. In the past, there were
areas where the average list size was above 2500, and in these
'designated' areas special inducements are available to encourage more doctors to practise there. This method of evening out
the spread of general practitioners has been effective in that
about two thirds of districts have average list sizes between
1900 and 2100.

(15) There are special arrangements for dealing with the problems of
rural areas (where doctors have at least 10% of their patients
living at least three miles from the main surgery) and Scottish
islands.

(16) There is a system of three years' required postgraduate *vocational
training* for general practitioners involving two years spent
working in the relevant hospital specialties and one year in a
training general practice selected for its high standards. A
trainer's fee is payable to the general practitioners who are
selected to act as trainers, and the payment to the trainee is
reimbursed by the NHS to the practice which employs the trainee
for a year. Medical students also receive at least four weeks
training in general practice during their undergraduate course.
There are additional courses for continuing postgraduate training
for practising doctors.

(17) General practitioners usually have *open access* to nearly all

hospital investigations, including some of the more sophisticated imaging techniques.

(18) General practitioners can write *prescriptions* for nearly all medicines which are available in the UK.

(19) *Visiting specialists,* such as psychiatrists, paediatricians, rheumatologists and so on, may hold regular (perhaps every two weeks) outpatient clinics in health centres and sometimes in other general practitioner premises. It is also possible for a general practitioner to arrange for a hospital specialist to see a patient at the patient's home to give an expert opinion. This is helpful for patients who are unable to travel to hospital to see a specialist. The cost of these domiciliary consultations is paid by the NHS.

Advantages of the UK general practitioner system

(1) Each patient has a *personal doctor* freely available to give continuing care to the patient and family over a long period (about ten years on average). The general practitioners, who depend on the patients registering with them for their income, tend to stay in the area, with their patients, for long periods.

(2) The *doctor has greater independence* and has the *responsibility* for the medical care of the patient. The NHS has only the responsibility for providing the overall framework for the system of care, the costs (raised indirectly from insurance and taxation of the general public) and maintenance of standards.

(3) *Referral to hospital* by the general practitioner can avoid unnecessary usage of hospitals and also ensure that the full medical history is passed on to the hospital doctors. Transfer of the medical records from general practitioner to general practitioner enables maximum usage of the information contained in the past medical history.

(4) Whilst providing free open access to general practitioners for the total population, the system also encourages *competition* between general practitioners (because of the capitation payments).

(5) There is an *even distribution of doctors* throughout the country with special allowances for the difficult rural areas.

(6) The arrangements for postgraduate and continuing *education* of general practitioners help to raise their standards and status. Most illnesses can be dealt with adequately (or better) in general practice, thus avoiding unnecessary hospital treatment.

The Government's *1987 White Paper on Primary Health Care* proposes changes to the existing system which can mostly be grouped into suggestions for modifications which cover three main areas:

(1)   the difficulties of practice in inner city areas (see Chapter 6, p. 111 et seq)
(2)   improvements in ways of maintaining standards and increasing consumer choice
(3)   increasing the emphasis on health promotion and preventive medicine in general practice

REFERENCES AND FURTHER READING

Abel-Smith B. (1976). *Value for Money in Health Services*. London: Heinemann Educational Books.

Allsop J., May A. (1986). *The Emperor's New Clothes. Family Practitioner Committees in the 1980s*. London: King Edward's Hospital Fund for London.

Cronin A. J. (1937). *The Citadel*. London: Gollancz.

Honigsbaum F. (1979). *The Division in British Medicine*. London: Kogan Page.

Secretaries of State for Social Services, England, Wales, Northern Ireland and Scotland (White Paper on Primary Health Care, Cmnd. 249; 1987). *Promoting Better Health. The Government's Programme for Improving Primary Health Care*. London: HMSO.

Stevens R. (1966). *Medical Practice in Modern England*. New Haven: Yale University Press.

Chapter

2

Education and Training for General Practice

**THE PLACE OF PRIMARY CARE WITHIN A MEDICAL SERVICE
• THE DOCTOR'S ROLE IN PRIMARY CARE • EDUCATION AND
TRAINING: THE CONTRIBUTION OF PRIMARY CARE • THE
PREREGISTRATION YEAR • VOCATIONAL TRAINING •
CONTINUING EDUCATION AND TRAINING • CONCLUSION**

Responsibility for maintaining health and for coping with illness lies first and last with individuals and those closest to them. When they feel unable to cope without help, they seek it from medical services. Less frequently, help is offered even when it has not been sought, e.g. in the immunization of children. Such health services as clean water and food are not the responsibility of the individual, but of the state.

In this country, there is a clear distinction between those services to which people in trouble have direct access (pharmacists, general practitioners, community nurses, dentists, opticians and hospital casualty services) and those which are reached only through referral from these primary carers. So primary medical care is distinguished from secondary above all because of this difference in *access*, but there is also an essential difference in *range*; primary services are relatively broad and general, secondary services relatively restricted and specialized. In this country, each is dependent on the other; good care increasingly requires cooperation and the sharing of responsibility between these two main elements in the total service.

This chapter is about education and training, but it is impossible to consider either without first addressing the question: *education and training for what role, what task?* For this reason, some description of primary care, particularly the way in which it concerns medical students, will precede the main subject.

It is not possible to consider preparation for primary care without considering preparation for medicine as a whole. The undergraduate stage, together with the preregistration year, form a stem common to all future medical careers and much of the basic knowledge, skill and experience gained during that time is relevant and useful to every branch. This common stem later creates a valuable background for mutual understanding and cooperation.

Education *and* training – these two words appear in the title and in this introduction, when it might seem that either alone would have been sufficient. But each represents an important strand that has to be intertwined with the other, especially during the undergraduate period. It was possible in the past to undergo a training for a role in medicine in the reasonable belief that it would last a lifetime; for such a training, the learning of facts by heart, imitation and the acceptance of authoritative experience from lectures, textbooks or ward rounds were appropriate additions to clerking patients. In the last fifty years, however, it has become increasingly obvious that *change* is a major characteristic of medicine – whether in new techniques, new ways of thinking, new attitudes in patients and colleagues, or even new diseases. All this makes a once-for-always preparation inappropriate; much of what one learns today will need to be replaced, even within ten years. So the aim of the medical teacher, especially in the undergraduate period, must be to educate doctors so that they are able to cope with a changing future. This requires methods familiar in other departments of universities but not sufficiently used in medicine in the past: less rote-learning, more thinking through new problems by the student; less dogma, more discussion; less certainty, more acceptance of the provisional quality of any truth.

Despite this difficult requirement for education to accommodate a changing future, training for the first job is also needed. House officers need certain facts and certain skills: they have to decide and act, to provide safe care under supervision and to feel secure in themselves while they continue to learn by doing.

So, education and training are not the same but they are both needed; that is why both words will continue to appear in this chapter.

The chapter will follow this sequence:

(1) (a) The place of primary care within a medical service.
    (b) The doctor's role in primary care.
(2) (a) The education and training of medical students and the contribution of primary care to this.
    (b) Specific postgraduate preparation.
    (c) Continuous learning.

THE PLACE OF PRIMARY CARE WITHIN A MEDICAL SERVICE

An ideal medical service aims to provide *care, cure, prevention* and *education*. Care and cure must be within easy reach and available when needed. The service must ensure that a great variety of different needs are recognized and sorted, so that they can be dealt with appropriately: minor problems do not require major interventions; major ones must be identified quickly if they are to receive the right expertise and have the earliest chance of help.

Although in some countries an attempt has been made to provide care on a totally specialized basis, this country has continued to provide its people with direct access to a service which is *general* at the point of entry, broad in scope and not specialized. It is significant that two of the countries which moved furthest towards first-line specialist care – Sweden and the USA – are both now trying to reverse this policy.

The division of medicine into specialist branches has been a necessary response to the great expansion in knowledge and techniques which medicine owes mainly to developments in the basic sciences. *Specialization* has brought great benefits to ill people, but also some disadvantages to them. Their problems are by no means always isolated – older patients especially bring multiple problems to doctors which cross specialist boundaries – and multiple specialist consultations are confusing, expensive in time and money, and often unnecessary. It is difficult for a specialist to keep a balanced and informed view of medicine outside his particular area of interest. Direct access to specialists adds the disadvantage that the patient has to choose the right person to consult first; for dental trouble this is easy, for abdominal pain very difficult. If, on the other hand, access to specialist services is only through *referral*, this difficulty is avoided; the interests and independence of patients are protected and specialists are more likely to receive the problems that they are best qualified to deal with.

Paradoxically, as specialization has increased, the need for a general doctor has become increasingly obvious in every country. In our own country, the number and distribution of general practitioners have been strictly controlled; there are very few people for whom a general doctor is not within easy reach. The system of referral and referral back is accepted and implemented by patients, specialists and general practitioners alike. *Primary care* is the aspect of medicine which most people experience most often – it forms the central element in our system and the general practitioner plays an essential role within it.

Table 2.1   *Consultation in the community by type of doctor, UK 1972–82*

Type of consultation	Per cent of consultations					
	1972	*1974*	*1976*	*1978*	*1980*	*1982*
NHS general practitioner	94	95	95	95	94	94
Private general practitioner	1	1	1	1	1	1
Specialist	2	2	1	2	3	2
Other	3	2	2	2	2	2

Source: General Household Surveys (1982).

THE DOCTOR'S ROLE IN PRIMARY CARE

A general practitioner accepts continuing responsibility in illness and health for a defined list of people who have chosen him or her for this purpose (on average, 2000 people).

In illness, it is in fact rare for a person to consult any doctor without first attempting some form of *self-help* or without discussing their trouble with someone else. Two out of three episodes of illness or injury are endured without reference to any medical service other than the pharmacist (most, but not all, of these episodes are of course minor or transient). Once consulted, however, the doctor's role in family care can still be described in words which come from the distant past and apply to all doctors or nurses: 'To cure sometimes, to relieve often, to comfort always' – to which must be added 'to prevent when possible'.

In primary care, the first and most frequent task is *assessment*. This word is more appropriate than 'diagnosis' because that implies identifying a disease. Not all of the problems that need to be identified in general practice can be called diseases without distorting reality – for

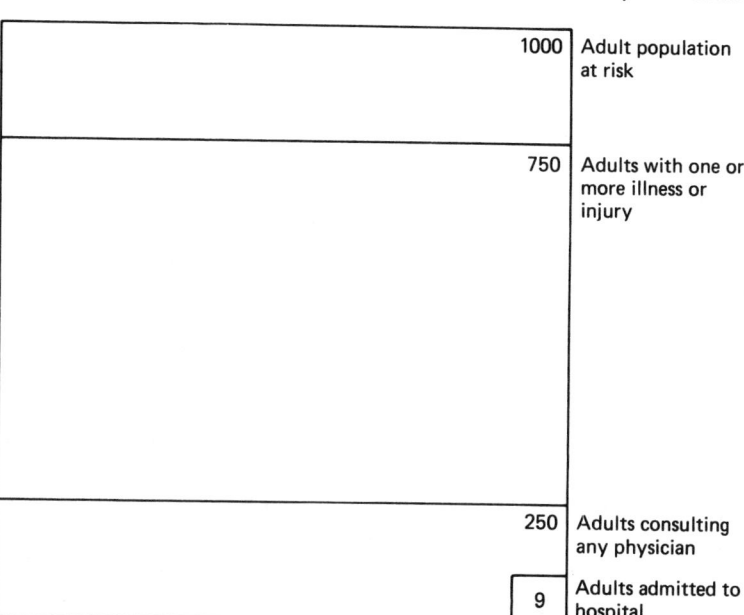

In any one month:

1000	Adult population at risk
750	Adults with one or more illness or injury
250	Adults consulting any physician
9	Adults admitted to hospital

Figure 2.1 Prevalence of illness and utilization of medical resources among 1000 adults.
Source: White et al. 1961 (after Horder and Horder 1954).

example, conflict between husband and wife or between parent and child, loneliness in the old or anxieties about physical sensations which prove groundless. General practitioners must be open to a very wide range of problems: many prove to be within the normal range of life experiences; many are those of subjective experience in a patient without objective evidence to substantiate the disorder of function or structure which is present; many can be recognized as nameable diseases with objective evidence of pathology. There are many more minor problems than major but the one sort can change into the other, making reassessment a constant concern. So assessment has to ask such questions as: What sort of problem? How many? Which matters most? Which need attention first? Can I cope myself or do I need help? Does the patient understand what the problem is?

While assessment is the doctor's first concern, patients are more likely to be anxious about the *management* of their problem and the outlook for the future. In this country, general practitioners assess and manage unaided about 90% of the problems that patients bring to them, but for the other 10% they may need a great variety of helpers – members of their own team on the spot, specialists in many branches of medicine, social services, voluntary services.

While hospital care is, for obvious reasons, most often short-term, the effective treatment of many acute disorders has given chronic and recurring diseases greater prominence, and this makes care while at home and at work increasingly important. Management in primary care often needs to be prolonged over a number of years; for such patients, personal continuity of doctors and nurses offers many advantages. The average length of contact between one general practitioner and one patient in this country is about 10 years.

Prevention is inseparable from assessment and management. For example, it may be possible to prevent the development of a complication of a disease, or the disability to which an injury might lead. However, prevention also includes helping people to recognize certain problems of which they are unaware, but which nevertheless affect health and can be helped. The most important of these is cigarette smoking, since this habit contributes to the cause of several life-threatening diseases. Twenty-five years ago few people would have been aware of this danger, or taken steps or sought help to avoid it. Doctors have been foremost in changing their own smoking habits and in influencing others to stop. Prevention may mean offering help and intervention where it has not been asked. If advice on smoking is one example, the detection of unsuspected raised blood pressure is another – this symptomless change being a threat to future health, yet controllable in many cases.

The term '*anticipatory care*' conveniently summarizes the continuing responsibility of general practice – a responsibility so exacting (all day, every day) that it must to some extent be shared with doctor partners, so wide that it must be shared with a team of other workers. But if people are to receive the personal doctoring that many have learnt to know and value, a large degree of *continuity* between one doctor and one patient is an important ingredient. Along with accessibility and the general, comprehensive and coordinating function already described, continuity makes it possible for a medical service to remain patient-centred while still providing the complex techniques that people and their diseases sometimes need.

What then are the qualities needed by general practitioners? A liking for people and a flair for diagnosis are central ones, but there will also need to be patience and tolerance, a preference for variety, the capacity to organize and a willingness both to accept responsibility and to share it. Primary care is probably not the best medical career for someone who finds personal relationships difficult, for those who particularly enjoy the manual skills of surgical work or who might be dissatisfied if intellectual problems are not always pursued to their logical conclusion.

EDUCATION AND TRAINING: THE CONTRIBUTION OF PRIMARY CARE

Before turning to education and training, it has been essential to outline the role and task at which these are directed, to define primary care and indicate the part which it plays in a larger whole, and to outline the role of the general practitioner in relation to other doctors and to other people who have a concern or responsibility in health and illness.

The period of basic, *undergraduate* education forms a common introduction to all of the many branches of medicine. It is not a special training for primary care – that comes later, just as training for a surgical career comes later.

If *secondary hospital care* still seems to dominate the clinical part of the basic curriculum, this is due partly to a long tradition and partly to the convenience of organizing teaching in one place where there is the greatest concentration of teachers and of patients with severe diseases which best illustrate disorders in the function and structure of the body. Until recently, medical students did not routinely experience medical care outside the hospital, where most illnesses are encountered and where other aspects of medicine can more easily be seen. A case can be made for basing a larger proportion of a curriculum in settings which would favour a more balanced programme, covering psychological, social and economic aspects of care, prevention and health promotion. Nevertheless, much of the undergraduate curriculum is of lasting relevance for doctors who enter a career in primary care.

General practice now contributes to undergraduate medical education in every university and school, but has been incorporated into curricula relatively recently and therefore has had to fit into an already established course of study which is mainly based on the pattern of organ or system divisions, relies largely on cases referred for hospital inpatient care, and is taught by those who have worked predominantly in that setting. The general practice contribution stretches across most of these divisions, forming a link between them. The range of cases seen by students while working in primary care corresponds far more closely to the actual incidence and prevalence of disorders in the community, with a predominance of less severe or earlier disorders.

During the total period of about a month when a student is attached to a general practitioner, there is a strict limit to the amount which can be learnt. Most students are impressed by the differences from their hospital experience rather than by the similarities, which are in fact greater. One of these differences is the wider *range* of problems; another is that new problems are seen *unselected* and as presented in the patient's own manner, relatively uninfluenced by previous medical contact. The familiarity of patient and doctor alters the consultation in a number of ways – for example, the ease with which anxieties are revealed or other members of the family involved. Many consultations enlarge on points raised at previous appointments, since repeat consultations in general practice are more easily arranged than at the hospital.

Students usually find it particularly interesting to observe how different doctors select their types of clientele, or how they deal in different ways with similar problems. Although the one-to-one contact of student with general practitioner is now a distinctive and valuable feature of this attachment, it is also important to see how at least one other general practitioner works; interesting contrasts can be seen.

Primary care does not, however, consist only in general medical practice. Students can learn much from nurses, health visitors, social workers, receptionists and pharmacists – and from patients, who often have revealing comments to make about their experience of illness, treatment, doctors and hospitals. None can explain better than the patient what it feels like to be ill with a particular disease, the way it threatens their life at work and at home, and how it affects their family. Such aspects are easily disregarded when teachers and students are concentrating on the objective aspects necessary to diagnosis and treatment.

If the attachment takes place close to final examinations, there are plenty of opportunities for the student to see and examine patients with physical problems of many kinds. It is, of course, an advantage if the student approaches the patients without any prior knowledge of their case, and it is often best to see them in their own home. There is no point, at this stage, however, in attempting to learn about practice organization or even about much of the detail of clinical management. It is far more important to sample the opportunities and limitations of this career, as one among the many choices open to the student in the future.

What then are the most important lessons to be learnt in the short time available out of a curriculum still based mainly in the hospital? I suggest that there should not be any attempt to train a future general practitioner; rather, the aim should be to gain a vision of medicine in the primary setting, where most people have most of their experience of medical care. This vision must include an impression of the range and distribution of problems which patients present to medical services; the opportunities for care, cure, prevention and education; the range of helpers and responses which can be brought to bear; thus, the growing importance of teamwork and the possibilities of referral in many directions (not only specialist medical referrals); and, within this setting, the need for a relationship with a personal medical adviser trained for a very broad scope, for the tasks of synthesis and coordination, and for long-term, continuing care. Relationship implies concern with, and respect for, individuality – including that of the student and of the doctor/teacher.

These seem to me to be some of the most essential among the many distinctive lessons to be learnt in primary care. Much of the rest is ground shared with more specialized teachers, in which primary carers can provide the opportunities for fitting different parts into a single picture of illness and care.

THE PREREGISTRATION YEAR

Some regard this year as an extension of the undergraduate period, before registration; others see it rather as the beginning of responsible practice. For most student doctors, the intense practical application of all they have learned, the chance to *do* rather than to watch, comes as a relief and an excitement, but there are also stresses – the pace of work; responsibility for other people, even though supervised by seniors;

close contact with ill people, especially if incurable or dying; long hours of work, with night duties; difficulties in working with other members of a large team.

Most preregistration jobs are in general medicine or general surgery, each lasting six months. At only one medical school (St Mary's Hospital Medical School) are preregistration appointments in general practice available.

The preregistration year is a time for developing *skills*, most of them already begun as a student, some scarcely experienced. Enhancing competence in clinical skills and judgement is the first priority – that is, solving problems and making decisions, especially about diagnoses. The familiar skills of interviewing and physical examination can be intensively practised, but the selection of appropriate investigations and treatments takes on a new urgency. So too does the need to relate to people in a way which creates open communication, trust and confidence. Other new challenges at this time include talking with relatives, working with other members of the medical, nursing and social work team, coping with unexpected behaviour whether in patients or colleagues, and thinking how to use limited resources wisely. It is at this stage also that the ethical and medico-legal issues can become matters of practical concern – for example, over the problem of informed consent, when a patient has to decide about undergoing an operation.

Registration takes place at the end of this year, conferring the theoretical right to practise and, in particular, the right to prescribe treatment without supervision. However, the newly registered doctor will not have had a special training for any branch of medicine. It would be impossible to practise in any part of the NHS (and unwise to set up in private practice) without further training.

Those who have already decided in favour of primary care will by now have considered how to enter a three-year vocational training scheme, but others will wish to keep their career options open; they will choose six-month appointments as senior house officers, until they decide in which direction they want to proceed (see Figure 2.2).

VOCATIONAL TRAINING

In the present state of the law, registration allows a doctor to practise unsupervised. Since 1981, however, the regulations of the NHS made it

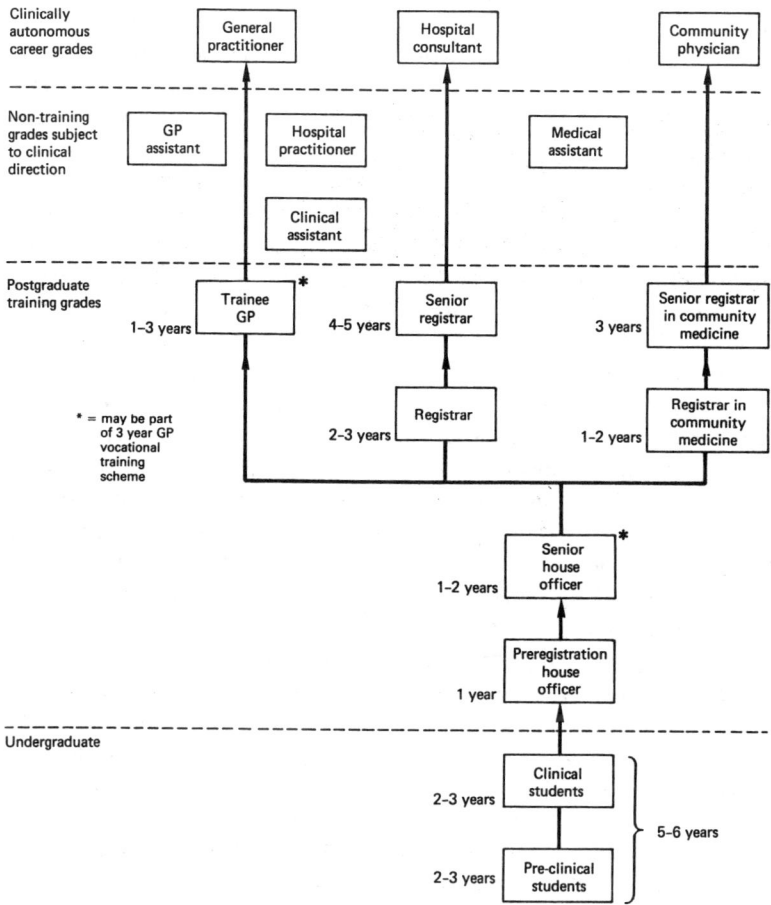

Figure 2.2 Medical career structure within the National Health Service. (Modified from Office of Health Economics (1984). *Compendium of Health Statistics.* London: HMSO, with permission.)

impossible to become a principal in general practice without undergoing three years of vocational training, partly in hospital posts, partly in a training practice and partly on courses. During this period, the doctor is earning and has responsibility for patients, under supervision.

The aim of this period is to train for *independent responsibility* as a general practitioner in primary care. Knowledge and skills already acquired have to be adapted and applied in new settings, such as the care of ill people in their own homes. New knowledge has to be gained – for example, about diseases or stages of diseases not seen in hospital practice, about preventive activities and health promotion, about working in a primary care team, or about the clinical and financial organization of a practice.

The detailed content of vocational training is described in a number of texts (see *References and Further Reading*). Their proposals are likely to exceed what is possible for any one person to achieve in a period that is inevitably occupied in part by the demands of the service in hospital, not all of which are relevant as training. Nevertheless, they are valuable as an ideal at which to aim, and as an indication of the wide range of knowledge and skills with which a fully-trained doctor must be sufficiently acquainted to recognize the limits of his or her own competence. No one can expect to be fully competent across the whole range; *teamwork* and *referral* are there to fill the gaps. Moreover, education and training do not cease at the end of this three-year period.

The content of vocational training is today partly determined by the examination for membership of the *Royal College of General Practitioners*, even though this – unlike the three years of training – is not obligatory. There is nevertheless considerable room for choice. It is well worth while using opportunities to strengthen areas of knowledge or experience recognized as weak – whether by choosing a combined training scheme or a particular hospital post which provides some missing experience, or by arranging a special attachment during the year in training practice.

This raises several important questions. How can you find out about training schemes? How do you choose and what is the procedure for application? What are the arrangements for living during this period if, for instance, you are married? Detailed guidance can be found elsewhere, but the fixed requirements are two years in a range of hospital posts with a large clinical commitment, one year in a practice selected for training, and a variable period in day or half-day release courses. There is a basic choice to be made between a three-year scheme as a pre-arranged sequence; or hospital posts and traineeship selected individually by the trainee and accepted by a postgraduate dean as suitable. For most people, the pre-arranged scheme is an easier and more appropriate choice, but at present there is strong competition for most of these schemes. In some places, it is possible for doctors with family commitments to train half-time, by doubling the length of the appointment.

Some schemes offer a variable choice of hospital posts, some a fixed sequence. Most offer a small choice of training practices with a named trainer. There is much to be said in favour of applying for schemes in the region where one might wish eventually to settle, because this may help in the subsequent problem of finding a practice.

In so far as there is choice in the selection of hospital posts, the availability of a good library can usually be assumed, but two other points are worth bearing in mind. First, as regards hospital posts, you should consider your own need for a particular subject or specialty. For most people, paediatrics, psychiatry and obstetrics/gynaecology are essential, followed closely in importance by general medicine – possibly combined with geriatrics – even though this may have been taken in the preregistration year. Training in smaller subjects is easier to acquire later than is training in these major ones. A second important consideration concerns the interest of the consultants in training future general practitioners and in devoting a proportion of their limited time to discussion of problems.

Good general practitioner trainers are often known through hearsay. What matters most is the enthusiasm for their work and their willingness to give time for discussion, both regularly and when needed urgently, as well as practical support if necessary. Regular review of the trainee's progress is another feature of good trainers.

Trainees should expect to spend between two thirds and three quarters of their time in seeing patients, devoting the rest to training sessions. They should be in a position to work more slowly than they may subsequently feel obliged to do as principals. All training schemes offer day or half-day release programmes, although the duration and pattern varies considerably. Programmes are usually decided in part by trainees in their local group.

As mentioned previously, the examination for Membership of the Royal College of General Practitioners is not obligatory, but at a time when competition for entry to practices is intense, it is in fact taken by most trainees. There are many revision courses available to help. The examination not only serves as an appropriate focus to test successful acquisition of training up to this point, but also, of course, constitutes the first contact with a College which the doctor can contribute to and benefit from in the future.

The importance of both vocational training and the Royal College may today be more obvious to those who were general practitioners before either existed than it is to younger doctors. The older ones can remember the isolation of many of their predecessors, the lack of development or change in their knowledge, and the loss of interest, enthusiasm and confidence, all of which often contrasted strongly with the experience of their colleagues in other branches of the profession.

Thus, continuing education has become an increasingly important feature of the general practitioner's life. The end of vocational training merely marks one further stage in a career-long process, but it may provide the best opportunity for a period of real contrast. Some doctors decide at this point to experience medicine in another country; they may be optimally equipped to do so and such experience is seldom a waste of time. However, this step does require confidence when there is anxiety about finding the right sort of practice in which to settle permanently, if that is their final intention.

CONTINUING EDUCATION AND TRAINING

Keeping up to date with new knowledge is not the only purpose of continuing education and training. Most mistakes in medical practice are due to a failure to *apply* what is known rather than to ignorance, and are likely to occur as a result of cutting corners or taking insufficient trouble, or through failing to communicate with other people who need to know. Whatever the field of medicine, there are influences that need to be countered if the doctor's best performance is to be maintained throughout a career. Experience may increase with age, but energy, enthusiasm, adaptability and self-criticism do not necessarily do so.

Regular contact with specialists contributes greatly to keeping up to date. Other needs are more likely to be provided by regular discussion with doctors who face the same clinical and organizational problems, in a process of *active learning* to which all can contribute. This needs to occur within a practice as well as in places more obviously designed for education, such as postgraduate centres.

Nothing is more likely to maintain enthusiasm and alertness of mind than reviewing performance, doing original research, writing, training students and postgraduates, or contributing to the organization of medical services or societies. It is paradoxical that giving out ideas is the best way of taking in and retaining them; active learning is more effective than passive. All doctors should, in some way, be teachers if they want to go on learning.

It is tempting to pursue those subjects which are of greatest interest to us and which, as a result, will become our strongest. We owe it to patients to seek out our areas of *weakness* and to devote at least some part of the available time to them.

Discussion with close colleagues is sometimes inhibited by a fear of revealing weakness or of hurting the feelings of another person. This may not seem relevant to continuing education if that is seen only as an intellectual process of gaining new knowledge. What ultimately matters, however, is the use of knowledge and the performance which results. Since the individual doctor increasingly needs to give service in the setting of a team, *communication* between team members is of the greatest importance; failure in this is now one of the most common reasons why things go wrong for patients. Communication is not just a matter of passing on information, important as that is. Success in a medical partnership or a primary care team is at the mercy of relationships; these can be open and sincere or they can be spoiled, sometimes wrecked, by undeclared resentments. It is not always too late or too difficult to discuss them. The importance of such situations – and the possibilities of dealing with some of them – is very obvious to those who undertake courses in management.

CONCLUSION

Medical education is a lifelong privilege. Relatively few people, other than doctors and nurses, are offered throughout their career a sequence of educational opportunities which can enrich their contributions to the welfare of others. Each stage builds on the previous stage, the first one rooted in what was learned long before a student enters medical school. The earliest stages have the greatest and most lasting influence. It is difficult later to undo what was originally learned, but knowledge is always provisional and sometimes proved to have been incorrect. Medicine remains an enjoyable career as long as the doctor maintains a constant process of renewal.

The nature and quality of a doctor's practice is determined as much by what the doctor brings to it as by the type of problems that patients present. Patients are always bringing new problems; education is always offering new ways of looking at them. The challenge is to go on *looking* and *listening*.

REFERENCES AND FURTHER READING

Ashbaugh D. G., McKean R. S. (1976). Continuing medical education. *J. Am. Med. Assoc.*, **236**, 1485.

British Medical Association (1984). *Handbook for Trainee Doctors in General Practice.* 2nd edn. London: BMA.

Freeling P. (1983). *A Workbook for Trainees in General Practice.* Bristol: John Wright.

Gray D. P. (1982). *Training for General Practice.* London: Macdonald & Evans Publications.

Hall M. S. (1983). *A General Practice Training Handbook, for Use by Trainers and Trainees.* London and Oxford: Blackwell Scientific Publications.

Harris C. M., Dudley H. A. F., Jarman B., Kidner P. H. (1985). Preregistration rotation including general practice at St Mary's Hospital Medical School. *Br. Med. J.*, **290**, 1797.

Horder J., Horder E. (1954). Illness in general practice. *Practitioner*, **173**, 177.

Office of Population Censuses and Surveys (1984). *General Household Survey 1982.* London: HMSO.

Royal College of General Practitioners (1984). *Combined Reports on Prevention.* Reports from General Practice Nos. 18–21. London: RCGP.

White K. L., Williams F. T., Greenberg B. G. (1961). The ecology of medical care. *New Engl. J. Med.*, **265**, 885.

3

Social and Economic Factors in Ill Health

DIMENSIONS OF INEQUALITIES IN HEALTH ● MODELS OF HEALTH ● SOCIAL AND ECONOMIC FACTORS IN THE AETIOLOGY OF ILL HEALTH ● POLICY IMPLICATIONS OF HEALTH INEQUALITIES

Health and ill health are not equally distributed. Mortality and morbidity rates vary in systematic ways. This chapter is concerned with how these inequalities in the health of different social groups can be explained, and in particular with the role of social and economic factors. In the first section, the major dimensions of inequality in health are briefly described; in the second, different models of health and their implications for modes of explanation are discussed; and in the third, the role of social and economic factors in the aetiology of ill health is considered.

DIMENSIONS OF INEQUALITIES IN HEALTH

The interrelationships between *health* and *social class* have been extensively studied. Peter Townsend, a sociologist and one of the authors of the Black Report on *Inequalities in Health*, has recently argued that:

'. . . social class must not be regarded as just another social indicator, like employment status, tenure, race or overcrowding, but as *the* social concept which is fundamental to the explanation of the distribution of health – to which the listed indicators are secondarily related.'

Although there is no general agreement about the meaning of social class, as used by Townsend it refers to the ranking of people in a society according to their social *and* economic position – their life chances broadly conceived. Various measures of social class are used in research, the most common being occupation, and the Registrar General's classification is the most frequently used in the health field to classify occupations into social classes. There are, of course, many difficulties associated with this and most other existing occupation-based measures of social class. Such measures do not, for example, differentiate as well between women's occupations as they do between men's, and it is difficult to classify certain groups – notably, married women without employment, the long-term unemployed, the retired etc. More generally, whilst occupation is a relatively good measure of many aspects of social and economic circumstances and life chances, there are some aspects that are not covered when social class status is reduced to occupation, as we shall see. Nevertheless, the picture that emerges from mortality and morbidity in different occupational social classes is one of great inequality.

Perhaps the most telling measure of these inequalities is *life expectancy*. One estimate suggests, for example, that a child born into occupational social class I can expect to live between five and seven years longer than one born into class V. For most causes of death, the lower the occupational class considered, the higher are the mortality rates. The gap is greatest during the first year of life. In 1985, for example, the infant mortality rate in occupational social class V was over twice as high as that in class I. During adult life, the gap is greater at younger ages than at older ages.

There are important exceptions to this general picture. For some causes of death, the gradient between the classes only holds for one sex. Deaths from all causes of cancer, for example, are fairly evenly spread amongst women in different social classes. In some specific instances the gradient is even reversed, as is the case with breast cancer deaths. However, some diseases – referred to as *diseases of affluence* – which have previously shown reverse gradients, for example non-valvular heart diseases, peptic ulcers and some cancers, are no longer exceptions to the general rule of higher mortality in lower occupational classes.

Overall, then, the picture is one of a considerable excess of premature deaths amongst people in lower occupational classes compared with higher classes. The scale and significance of this is powerfully depicted in the following quote from the Black Report:

'If the mortality rate for class I had applied to classes IV and V during 1970–72 . . . 74 000 lives of people aged under 75 would not have been lost. This estimate includes 10 000 children and 32 000 men of working age.'

More recent data for mortality over the period 1972–82 published in August 1986 confirm that the general picture has not changed; indeed, the gap between the mortality rates in higher and lower social classes may actually have widened during the decade concerned, although this interpretation is the subject of considerable controversy.

These inequalities in mortality are paralleled by similar inequalities in *morbidity*. According to the latest data for 1984 from the government sponsored annual *General Household Survey*, 9% of men and women in the professional socio-economic group* reported a long-standing condition which limited their activity in some way, compared with 24% of men and 34% of women in the unskilled group.

Occupational social class is not the only factor determining health inequality. In all occupational classes and at all ages, *males* are on average about 60% more likely than *females* to die prematurely. However, with regard to many aspects of morbidity, especially those not associated with life-threatening conditions, the pattern for men and women is reversed. For example, in 1984 amongst people aged between 16–44 years, 9% of men and 12% of women reported some restricted activity due to illness in the 14 days before the interview. Similarly, in the same age group, the average number of days on which illness restricted normal activity in the non-manual socio-economic group was 12 for men compared with 18 for women, and in the manual group it was 16 for men compared with 19 for women. Also, women are diagnosed as suffering from psychiatric disorders approximately three times as frequently as are men.

For many years, married people have been found to have better health than those who are not married. Since the 19th century, mortality rates have been lowest for the married, higher for the single and highest of all for the widowed and divorced. The interaction of the

---

*The General Household Survey uses a measure of social class usually referred to as *socio-economic groups*, as opposed to the Registrar General's *occupational social class*. The two classifications are, however, largely comparable.

different dimensions of health inequality is also apparent, for amongst married people men have a higher mortality rate than women, and those in lower social classes have a higher mortality rate than those in higher social classes. Rates of self-reported illness, of mental illness and of other measures of morbidity, are also related to *marital status* in a similar way, although these data are much more limited.

Mortality and morbidity rates also vary *geographically*. Since at least the last century, for example, standardized mortality ratios have been found to be higher in the northern regions – notably Scotland, Ireland and the north-east of England – than in the southern regions, and the same distribution is apparent for many facets of morbidity. Similarly, there is a strong association between the degree of urbanization and ill health. Once again, the overlapping nature of inequalities in health is evident. Whilst in each region the social class gradient in mortality rates persists, people in each occupational social class in the northern regions have a higher mortality rate than those in the same class in the south of the country.

Information on inequalities in health in different *ethnic groups** is extremely limited. This is partly due to the difficulties involved in producing a workable and acceptable classification of ethnic groups, but also is a reflection of the way in which the health problems of black minority ethnic groups have been defined.

Medical research and health service provision have tended to be preoccupied with conditions such as rickets, osteomalacia, thalass-aemia, sickle-cell anaemia and tuberculosis. However, whilst these conditions are undoubtedly important, they affect an *extremely* small number of people and do not appear to be the major health problems facing black ethnic minority groups. The evidence suggests that these are the same as those experienced by other sections of the community. A recent study in a predominantly white general practice population indicated that respiratory infections, skin disorders and psycho-emotional problems were the most prevalent. A phone-in health

---

*There is considerable and at times acrimonious debate about the use of the terms *ethnicity* and *race*. The former, it is argued, is a social label and therefore better than race which implies a biological basis for group differences. Such a basis has no support from genetic research. The term ethnicity, however, is considered to be too closely tied to ideas of cultural differences, neglecting the significance of 'racial' discrimination on the basis of skin colour or religion, for example.

counselling service provided for a predominantly Asian community found that a high percentage of calls were similarly concerned with respiratory problems, mental health and skin complaints.

Although limited, the evidence available does indicate important differences in the amount, rather than the kind, of ill health experienced by different ethnic groups. Adult mortality in first generation black migrant groups is lower than that for the white majority population in Britain, a pattern which reflects a 'healthy migrant' effect. However, this health advantage is not carried over to the next generation born in this country. Babies of women born in the UK, for example, have lower perinatal and infant mortality rates than babies whose mothers were born in the Indian subcontinent or the West Indies, whilst babies of women born in Pakistan have high mortality rates. It is also important to note that, contrary to the situation prevailing in the white majority population, female death rates are higher than those for males amongst migrant groups. Similarly, a small scale study of the annual incidence of tuberculosis found that it was three per 100 000 amongst white children, 63 amongst British-born Asian children, and 114 for Asian children born outside the UK; it appeared that the majority of these cases were contracted in the UK.

Some black ethnic minority groups are also more likely to be diagnosed as mentally ill than the majority white population. West Indians born outside the UK, for instance, were found in one study to be more than 3.5 times as likely to be admitted to a mental hospital suffering from schizophrenia than the British-born population. In contrast, however, Asians have lower rates of mental disturbance, suicide or mental hospital admission than any other black minority ethnic group or the white population.

Whilst the UK data on ethnic variation in health are extremely limited, they are consistent with patterns of inequality documented more extensively in other countries. In the USA, for example, the mortality rate amongst black people is 33% higher than amongst white people and 90% higher with regard to infant mortality.

These then are the major dimensions of inequalities in health in Britain today. That they exist is not denied, but the reasons for them are controversial. They have been described only very briefly here and are discussed in much greater detail elsewhere (see *References and Further Reading*).

MODELS OF HEALTH

Interpretation depends largely on the model of health that is adopted. Today, a *bio-medical model* of ill health is generally accepted. This model portrays diseases as having specific causes, such as microbial agents, hormone deficiencies, genetic factors or physiological stress. Flowing from this model is the concept of health as a virtue and largely a question of individual responsibility in terms of life-style and health care. Ill health is seen to be either a misfortune or a result of an individual's irresponsibility. One extreme example of this particular position appeared in an article in the *British Medical Journal* in 1978. This article reported the results of a study of 250 deaths amongst hospital patients aged under 50 years conducted by the Medical Services Group of the Royal College of Physicians. The authors concluded that:

'no fewer than 98 patients contributed to their own death through overeating, drinking, smoking and not complying with treatment,'

and they labelled these as cases of *self-destruction*. Another more recent example of this approach to understanding contemporary patterns of health and ill health is the following statement made in 1986 by Edwina Currie, Junior Minister for Health, concerning the cause of the high mortality and morbidity rates in the north of England:

'I honestly don't think that the problem has anything to do with poverty . . . the problem very often for people is, I think, just ignorance . . .'

The bio-medical model of health and illness has undoubtedly led to considerable theoretical and medical advances. To criticize it is not to deny this, nor to argue that all modern medicine can be represented in such a consistent and clear-cut manner. Rather, it is to suggest that there are, in fact, very few diseases for which a bio-medical model has provided a complete explanation, and that to gain a fuller understanding we must look beyond this model's narrow confines. An alternative approach is provided by what is often referred to as the *social model* of health and disease. This model was somewhat paradoxically embraced by Rudolf Virchow whose work on cellular pathology contributed a great deal to the development of the bio-medical model. It was, however, the same Virchow who argued that:

'Medicine is a social science and politics nothing more than medicine on a large scale.'

In the social model, health is conceived as an interactive relationship between the body, the mind and the environment within the context of historical and individual biographical time. According to this model, as Nicky Hart – a medical sociologist – has recently argued,

'Medically defined disease categories are the end-products of a process in which social inequalities and powerlessness, exposure to critical life events, personal vulnerability factors and coping responses coalesce to produce a positive or negative disease outcome.'

Coming from such a social model is the belief that differences in the health experiences of different social groups are created and shaped by the way our society is structured. These differences, it is argued, reflect the unequal distribution of control over, and therefore access to, the social and economic resources human beings depend on for their survival and well-being.

SOCIAL AND ECONOMIC FACTORS IN THE AETIOLOGY OF ILL HEALTH

Obviously, there can be no simple explanation for the complex pattern of health inequalities briefly described above. It is beyond dispute that factors associated with individual behaviour, such as smoking and diet, play an important part, but it is equally self-evident that these will interact with other social and economic factors over which individuals have little if any control. As the authors of the Black Report argued:

'. . . There is undoubtedly much which cannot be understood in terms of the impact of specific factors, but only in terms of the more diffuse consequences of the class structure: poverty, working conditions and deprivation in its various forms.'

In the remainder of this chapter, we will look briefly at some of the most important dimensions of social and economic inequalities in contemporary Britain.

Poverty and health inequalities

One of the most important aspects of deprivation from a health perspective is the nature and distribution of poverty. There is, in fact, considerable debate about how poverty should be defined, a debate which has a long history. One of the most famous studies of poverty was that undertaken in York in 1899 by Seebohm Rowntree. Rowntree argued that families whose 'total earnings were insufficient to obtain the minimum necessaries for the maintenance of merely physical efficiency', were experiencing primary poverty. He defined this poverty line by estimating the average nutritional needs of adults and children, and translating these into quantities of food and then cash equivalents. He then added sums for other essential items such as clothing and heating, varying these for households of different sizes.

Today's social security benefits, paid by the Department of Health and Social Security (DHSS), are still essentially based on such a *subsistence* view of poverty, although they are increased annually. Regulations define the items of normal day-to-day living that families are expected to meet from basic *supplementary benefit*.* Apart from housing costs (which are met from housing benefit) these items include:

'. . . in particular: food; household fuel; the purchase, cleaning, repair and replacement of clothing and footwear; normal travel costs; weekly laundry costs; miscellaneous household expenses, such as toilet articles, cleaning materials, window cleaning; the replace-ment of small household goods (for example, crockery, cutlery, cooking utensils, light bulbs); and leisure and amenity items, such as television licences and rental, newspapers, confectionery and tobacco.'

The level of supplementary benefit provides one way of drawing the line below which people can be said to be living in poverty in the UK today, although there is considerable evidence that supplementary benefit does not provide sufficient money to meet even these basic needs. There are, however, other ways of defining poverty. Notable here is the work of Peter Townsend, who has argued that poverty is:

'. . . the absence or inadequacy of those diets, amenities, standards, services and activities which are common or customary in society. People are deprived of the conditions of life which ordinarily define membership of society.'

If such a *relative* definition of poverty is accepted as more fitting to the 1980s, it is still necessary to decide what level of resources would be necessary to allow people to live 'as is common and customary in

---

*The social security system has undergone extensive changes, as a result of the *1986 Social Security Act*, which were implemented in April 1988. Supplemen-tary benefit has been the major *means-tested benefit*, but this was eventually replaced with another called income support. In addition to means-tested benefits there are a range of *National Insurance benefits*, receipt of which is dependent on the payment of National Insurance contributions.

society'. In his 1969 study of poverty in the UK, Peter Townsend constructed a provisional *index of relative deprivation* using twelve summary measures of the style of living customary in society at that time. These included not having had a holiday away from home in the last 12 months and not having had an afternoon or evening out for entertainment in the last two weeks, as well as more widely accepted indicators such as having no refrigerator, no sole use of four basic indoor amenities (a flush toilet and a washbasin, for example), and not having a cooked meal on one or more days in the past fortnight. He then calculated that level of income below which the risk of experiencing one or more of these dimensions of deprivation increased rapidly, arriving at a figure of 150% of the supplementary benefit level.

Townsend's index has been criticized because the list of indicators he used was arbitrary, and because people may lack one or more of the elements through choice rather than shortage of money. In 1983, however, data from a survey conducted by Market and Opinion Research International (MORI) allowed an index to be constructed on the basis of what people in Britain actually feel to be 'necessary and which all adults/families should be able to afford and which they should not have to do without.' The items included in this index of relative deprivation closely resemble those in Townsend's, and are illustrated in Table 3.1 below. The figure also shows that proportion of the sample who felt that the item was 'necessary'. According to further analysis of the data collected by MORI in 1983, the risk of being unable to afford one or more of these items increased significantly below an income equivalent to 133% of the supplementary benefit level.

For these and a number of other reasons, an income level of up to 140% of the level of supplementary benefit is widely accepted as an indicator of *low income*, even in official government surveys. People on incomes at this level are often described as *on the margins of poverty*, and data on the number of people living at these income levels are an indication of the number of people experiencing relative poverty.

How many people can be said to be poor in Britain today? The most recent data available are for 1983. In that year, there were 2 780 000 adults and children living on incomes below the level of supplementary benefit, 6 130 000 dependent on supplementary benefit, and a further 7 470 000 dependent on incomes up to 140% above the supplementary benefit level. This represents 15% of the population living on incomes at or below the official poverty standard and a total of 31% of

Table 3.1 *Market and Opinion Research International/London Weekend Television Index of Deprivation, 1983*

Item	% of sample describing these items as 'necessary'
Heating to warm living areas	97
Public transport for one's needs	88
A warm waterproof coat	87
Three meals a day for children	82
Two pairs of all-weather shoes	78
Toys for children	71
Celebrations on special occasions, like Christmas	69
Roast joint or equivalent once a week	67
New, not second-hand, clothes	64
Hobby or leisure activity	64
Meat or fish every other day	63
Presents for friends/family once a year	63
Holidays away from home for one week a year	63
Leisure equipment for children (bicycles etc.)	57

The survey from which these data are drawn involved a representative quota sample of 1174 people aged 16 years and over, interviewed at home in eighty sampling points across Great Britain.
Source: Table 4, Lansley and Weir (1983).

the population in or on the margins of poverty. The latter figure compares with 28% in 1981, and it is probable that since 1983 the proportion in or on the margin of poverty will have continued to increase.

It is important to try to gain some understanding of what these income levels mean. In 1986, it was estimated that for a married couple, the higher long-term rate of supplementary benefit (available to everyone who has been on benefit for more than a year, except for the unemployed) was worth only 40.3% of average net earnings. *But what do these incomes signify in health terms?* The index of relative deprivation in Table 3.1 illustrates the types of things people on these incomes will be deprived of; obviously, the lower the income the more items people will be unable to afford.

The effects of poverty on health will, therefore, be many and varied. Shortage of money will affect the general environment in which people live, not only in relation to housing standards but also in terms of the physical environment surrounding the home, for example the availability of play space for children, the proximity of dangerous roads and exposure to atmospheric pollution. Poverty will also affect the food that people are able to eat, the clothes they wear, their ability to keep themselves warm in the winter and the opportunities they have available to them to lead a full and satisfying social life. Lack of money will also lead to considerable anxiety and stress, as people endeavour to make ends meet on inadequate incomes, and this too will have a detrimental effect on mental and physical health.

The greatest share of the financial resources of low income families goes on housing, fuel and food, leaving very little if anything to spare for clothing, outings and other items. Fuel costs in particular often prove to be too great a strain. In the year ending September 1986, for example, 130 000 household fuel supplies were disconnected because of fuel debts. More importantly perhaps, there has been a big increase in the number of households who are having sums deducted directly from their benefits to pay off arrears of fuel bills. When this happens it means families have much less money and less flexibility to meet day-to-day living expenses. Research has shown that poor families will try to make ends meet by cutting back on the most flexible items of expenditure, often food. Although this may not mean absolute shortages in most instances, the effects on diet can be extreme. It has been shown, for example, that the cost of the DHSS recommended diet for pregnant women is half of the total weekly benefit for a single person. A recent report from the London Food Commission concluded:

'Low income means less money available to spend on food . . . Supplementary benefit levels are totally inadequate for ensuring a healthy diet. The new social security system . . . is unlikely to improve the access of those on low incomes to good quality, reasonably priced food. . . .'

But who are the poor? Certain types of households are much more likely to be poor than others. Table 3.2 below shows the percentages of people living on incomes below 140% of the supplementary benefit level by the type of household they live in and by their employment status. It also shows the percentage of the total population in these household and employment groups. These figures illustrate how pensioners, people in one parent families and those in large families are particularly over-represented amongst the poor, as are the sick and disabled and the unemployed. The table also illustrates that although unemployment is the most important cause of poverty today, a quarter of people in paid employment are earning 'poverty wages'.

Two groups particularly at risk of experiencing poverty – *women* and minority *ethnic* groups – are not explicitly identified in Table 3.2. The scale of the problem women face is, however, reflected in the figures for one parent families and the elderly. In 1985, 14% of all families were headed by a lone parent, a proportion that has increased from 8% in 1971. Almost 90% of these lone parents are women, and in 1983 52% of all one parent families were receiving supplementary benefit compared with less than 10% of all two parent families. Altogether, 60% of families headed by a lone parent were living in or on the margins of poverty according to the definition discussed earlier, compared with 20% of two parent families. Similarly, women account for approximately 67% of all the elderly over 75 years old. Another group not explicitly identified in the table is *children*. In 1983, nearly one third of all children were living in or on the margins of poverty, and a quarter of these children were in one parent families.

The figures in Table 3.2 also assume that income is equally distributed within households, an assumption which restricts our understanding of women's experience of poverty. The distribution of material and other resources within households was, in fact, a focus of research interest in the early years of this century. In the report on his survey of poverty in York published in 1901, Seebohm Rowntree noted that:

> 'extraordinary expenditure . . . is met by reducing the sum spent on food. As a rule in such cases, it is the wife and sometimes the children who have to forgo a portion of their food – the importance of maintaining the strength of the wage-earner is recognized and he obtains his ordinary share.'

In more recent years, however, this issue has been relatively neglected in research on poverty, although during the 1970s some researchers did begin to shed light on the private sphere of the family, and they discovered that the same processes were still at work. In her study of large families in 1977, for example, Hilary Land noted that:

> 'The impact of a low income, bad housing and insufficient food is not borne equally by all members of the family. Resources are allocated by reference to custom or tradition and the interests of some members of the family are sacrificed to the interests of others. In particular, it is noticeable, that in many aspects, the mother of the family puts the needs of her husband and children before her own.'

Table 3.2 *Who are the poor? Data for Great Britain, 1983**

| | Household types | | | | Employment status groups | | | |
	Over pensionable age	Couples with children	One parent families	Single people	Full-time employed/ self-employed	Unemployed more than three months	Sick/ disabled	Others**
Percentage of those on incomes below 140% of supplementary benefit by household type and employment status	35%	34%	9.5%	15.6%	26%	21%	3.7%	25%
Percentage of total population in different household types and employment status groups	16.7%	43%	4.5%	17.6%	62.5%	7.64%	2.9%	10.3%

*These figures exclude the institutional population.

**The 'others' category amongst the employment status groups consists largely of lone parents, full-time students, full-time workers temporarily away from work (for reasons other than sickness) on part or no pay, persons looking after sick relatives, and others under pensionable age not working or not seeking work.

Source: DHSS (1986).

Unemployment and health inequalities

As noted above, unemployment has been one of the most important causes of the recent increase in the number of people living in or on the margins of poverty. After almost twenty years of full employment throughout the 1950s and 1960s, during which time the proportion of the labour force unemployed averaged around 1.6%, unemployment began to rise slowly at first and then with increasing speed. By 1979, there were 1.3 million people officially unemployed in Britain or 5.6% of the labour force, and by the end of 1986 this figure had increased to 3.3 million people, or 13% of the labour force. Over 40% of these people have been out of paid employment for more than a year, and over a quarter for more than two years. Fortunately, since the latter part of 1987 there has been a small reduction in the number of unemployed.

It is also important to note that official figures include only those people receiving benefit because of unemployment. They fail to include many people who are actively seeking work, but who are not entitled to benefit – particularly many married women, people on special government schemes and workers aged between 60 and 65 years who have been 'involuntarily' retired. One estimate suggests that a more accurate figure of the number unemployed would be about 10% more, and even this does not include a large number of women and older people who, though not actively seeking work, would take paid employment if a job were available.

As the unemployment level has risen, there has been increasing concern about the health implications. Attention has been directed at two key questions: *does unemployment affect health and, if so, how?* It is interesting to note that a similar controversy over the relationship between unemployment and health raged in the depression years of the 1930s.

Research from the 1930s and more recently shows beyond doubt that there is an association between unemployment and ill health. This is despite the fact that in some instances it is apparent that unemployment may lead to an improvement in the health of individuals (who are no longer exposed to particular physical or chemical hazards, for example). Mortality rates, and rates of limiting long-term illness, disability and psychological disturbance, have all been found to be higher amongst the unemployed than amongst the employed. There are, however, a number of alternative ways of explaining these associations.

The association between unemployment and ill health could be an *artefact*. It could be that the unemployed are 'exaggerating' their ill health – adopting the sick role – in order to avoid the stigma of unemployment in a society where to be unemployed, even during a depression, is seen to be in some way your own fault. Obviously, this explanation could not be applied to the higher than expected mortality rate amongst the workless, but there is some evidence that it could apply to other aspects of ill health amongst unemployed people.

A second possible artefactual explanation arises from the way in which unemployment is socially distributed. Of particular importance here is the relationship between unemployment and occupational *social class*. Unemployment is, in fact, proportionately much higher amongst workers in lower occupational social classes than amongst those in higher classes and, contrary to popular belief, as unemployment levels have risen this unequal distribution has become more rather than less pronounced. The average rate of unemployment during 1975–77 was 4% amongst professionals, managers and employers, compared with 18% amongst semi-skilled and unskilled manual workers. By 1983, the rate had increased to 6% in the former group compared with 32% amongst unskilled and semi-skilled workers.

Unemployment rates are also higher for *ethnic minority groups* than for the white majority population. In the spring of 1985, the unemployment rate amongst black minority groups was twice as high as that for the white population, and a third of all ethnic minority young people aged between 16 and 24 years were out of work, compared with 16% of the same age group in the white population.

Unemployed people, therefore, are disproportionately drawn from those social groups that are disadvantaged in health terms, and so it is to be expected that more ill health will be found amongst the unemployed than the employed.

Another possible explanation for the association between unemployment and ill health could be that ill health *causes* unemployment. It is argued that people who have poorer health will be more likely to lose their jobs and less likely to find jobs again when unemployed, and so it would be expected that the unemployed will have higher mortality and morbidity rates than the employed. There is evidence that such health-related selection may explain part of the excess ill health found amongst the unemployed: for example, people with a history of mental illness, or with a physical or mental disability, have more difficulty finding employment than the 'able-bodied'. In one large-scale government survey, only 53% of people who were registered as disabled had worked at some stage in a 12-month period following unemployment, compared with 83% of those with no health problems.

Under different economic conditions, different 'degrees' of ill health will be more or less likely to cause unemployment. The important question in the present context, however, is *how much* of a contribution does such a process make to the excess mortality and morbidity found amongst the unemployed – and how much, on the other hand, is attributable to the social and economic consequences of unemployment?

An important contribution to this debate is now being made by data from the Longitudinal Study (LS), in which a 1% sample of the total UK population drawn from the 1971 census is being followed. Early results from the LS show that *mortality* rates over the period 1971–5 for men seeking work at the time of the 1971 census were some 30% higher than that of the total LS sample. Even when taking account of the social class distribution of the unemployed, the excess mortality does not disappear. In seeking to explain this, the researchers on the LS considered in some detail the possibility that ill health might cause unemployment, but a recent paper concluded:

'Our results relating to the men seeking work in 1981 all point in the same direction as the results for 1971. The high mortality which we observe . . . appears not to be explained by either the pre-existing health of these groups or their socio-economic status prior to unemployment.'

Mortality rates of the wives of men seeking work at the time of the 1971 census were also found to be approximately 20% higher in the ten years following the census than the mortality rate of other married women in the sample. As noted, whilst it may be possible to argue that men are selected into unemployment due to health problems, it is much more difficult to make a case that these same men selected their wives on health grounds too.

Research from the Medical Research Council Social Psychology Unit at Sheffield Univesity has similarly shown that the excess *psychological illness* consistently found amongst unemployed people cannot be explained in terms of pre-existing mental illness, but rather, that some at least of this psychological distress is directly linked to the experience of unemployment.

Unemployment therefore appears to have direct adverse effects on mental and physical health, and we need to understand how this happens. An important distinction has to be made between the direct experience of unemployment and the effects of a *recession* on those in work (Figure 3.1). Looking first at unemployment per se, this figure suggests that the adverse effects on health may result from three related processes: psychological processes, an increase in health-damaging behaviour such as smoking, and/or deteriorating material living standards.

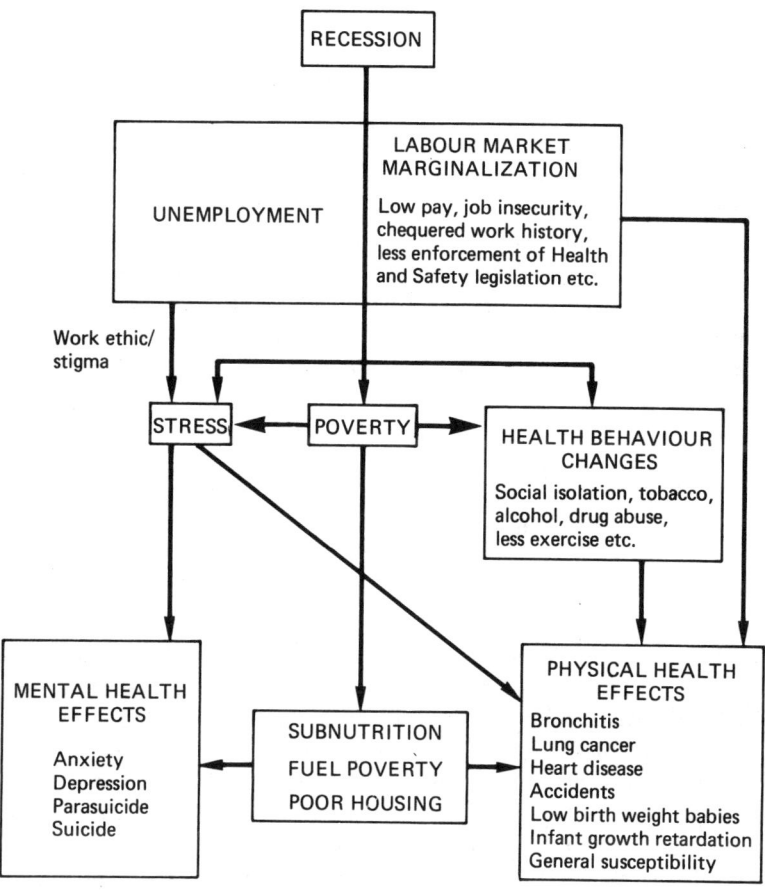

Figure 3.1 Possible pathways between the effects of recession and adverse health outcomes.
Source: Unemployment and Health Study Group (1986).

The relationship between poverty and unemployment has already been noted. Unemployment can have a dramatic effect on *income*. A DHSS study of unemployed men begun in 1978, for example, found that 45% of the sample were living on incomes which were less than half of those they had received when in employment. Similarly, long-term unemployed people have disposable incomes of around two thirds of the incomes of those in stable *but low paid* employment. The ways in which such incomes can adversely affect health have also been discussed, and studies looking specifically at the living standards of the unemployed confirm this general picture. One recent study, for example, found that one in four households with an unemployed person does not have enough money for a whole week's food.

Paid employment establishes an individual's personal identity, provides important social networks, a way of structuring time and is, perhaps, the single most important means whereby others assess an individual's social status. Closely tied to all of this is the fact that employment provides a 'legitimate' source of income – no matter how low – in contrast to receipt of means-tested benefits. Unemployment is therefore likely to be a stigmatizing, disruptive and isolating experience, and can cause considerable mental distress.

Only a few studies have considered the position of unemployed women. This work suggests that whilst the experience may be different, the financial and psychological effects can still be considerable. Researchers have also pointed to the similarities between the experience of unemployment for men and that of women at home looking after young children or other dependants, who have also been found to have above average rates of mental illness. More research is needed in this area.

The effects of unemployment within households has also been studied. One small scale study looked at the effects of unemployment on family relationships where the father was unemployed and there were young children in the household. These men did not necessarily become actively involved in domestic work and child care; instead, the women continued to take most of this responsibility and carried the additional burden of giving their partner emotional support, coping with the extra work their partner's presence created and managing a much reduced household budget. Such situations can be expected to affect adversely both the mental and physical health of women.

Children too can be adversely affected. There is little evidence of an association between child abuse and unemployment, but rates of admission to hospital are higher than expected amongst children with unemployed fathers, although it is not clear whether this reflects an increased incidence of illness or families' failure to cope with illness. Additionally, it would appear that parental unemployment may have long-term detrimental effects on children's growth and development.

There has been very little research on the impact of unemployment on demand for health services, but the study undertaken by the general practitioner Norman Beale and the statistician Susan Nethercott, illustrates the important contribution that general practice based research can make in this sphere. Beale and Nethercott studied the families of a group of 129 workers before and after the closure of a factory. They reported a significant increase in morbidity reflected in increased consultation rates amongst these workers, beginning two years before job loss, and argued that there was an increased work load and cost for the NHS directly attributable to a rising unemployment rate.

Given the evidence that unemployment has a direct effect on the mental and physical health of the unemployed and their families, the concentration of unemployment in lower occupational social classes and black minority ethnic groups noted above takes on a new significance. Unemployment is not a separate issue from social class or race but an integral part of the experience of being in lower social classes or being black. As such it can be expected to make a major contribution to the social, economic and psychological factors which adversely affect health in these classes and amongst black people.

The health of women

The different experience of men and women in relation to both mortality and morbidity was described at the beginning of this chapter, and in earlier sections some of the social and economic factors that can be expected to contribute to these differences have been discussed. There are, however, other factors which should be considered. Hilary Graham, a sociologist, has recently argued that:

'Differences in the health experiences of men and women, like differences between the social classes, are seen to reflect differences in the way that people live. In particular, sex differences are seen to reflect differences in the working conditions of men and women. In general terms, it appears that it is the particular kind and pace of men's work which makes men as a sex more vulnerable to premature death. Similarly, it is the kind and pace of work which women do which makes women more vulnerable to ill health.'

What, then, do we know about the kind and pace of work that women do? We know that they are expected to take the major responsibility for child care and domestic labour. Less well recognized is that part of domestic labour which involves the caring work that women do in providing for elderly, frail or dependent relatives and friends. These *nurturant role activities*, as they have been termed, are used to explain some part of the ill health experienced by women compared with men. Nurturant activities, it is suggested, prevent women from getting enough sleep generally and mean that they will be less well cared for themselves when they are sick. High levels of sleeplessness, fatigue, and social isolation are found amongst the mothers of young children, especially those without employment outside the home. Where housing conditions are poor, play areas for children inadequate, local transport and other facilities limited, it is women who bear a disproportionate share of the burden, because it is women who spend most time in the home and make most use of local facilities.

Further, as already noted, resources may not be equally distributed within the home. In many households, and not just those on low incomes, women do not have equal access to financial and other resources and do not have an equal say in the way that available money is spent. They may therefore be expected to meet items of expenditure, such as food, clothing, heating and in some cases housing, but have little – if any – control over how much of the household income they receive.

This unequal distribution of resources and power between men and women within households could explain the somewhat paradoxical findings from a survey of women in one and two parent families conducted recently by Hilary Graham. She found that, generally, women in one parent families were materially and socially worse off than women in two parent families, and they reported worse health. However, she also found that women caring for children alone often felt, and actually were, financially better off than women in low income, two parent families. She argues that this reflects the greater control that lone parents have over the resources coming into the home, albeit that these resources are very limited.

The health implications of the interaction between women's nurturant role and their involvement in the formal labour market have also been explored. One of the most significant social changes since the end of the second world war has been the increasing proportion of married women in the formal labour force. The proportion grew from one in ten in 1921, to one in two in 1981. During the 1980's, however, as a result of the recession, the proportion has remained fairly stable with six out of ten married women aged 16 to 59 years in employment in 1984. Whether or not married women work, and whether they work full time or part time, is closely linked to the age of their children. Only a quarter of women with a child under five years were in paid employment in 1982/1984, and 84% of them worked part time. In comparison, 64% of women with children over five were employed, 70% of whom worked full time.

There has been a great deal of research into the implications of married women's employment for the welfare of their children and, to a lesser extent, their partners. Their earnings were and still are widely seen as 'pin money' and their employment often considered to be irresponsible. Increasingly, however, it has been recognized that the financial contribution which married women make to household income is often vitally important in keeping the family above the poverty line. There are, in addition, a large number of one parent families with dependent children where women's earnings are the only source of income other than dependence on state benefits. Caring for children or others full time can be a lonely and isolating experience that society devalues. Employment outside the home, for women as well as for men, can therefore be an important source of social networks and personal identity, as well as a source of income.

Paid employment does, however, threaten the health of some women. When they are in the labour force, domestic responsibility and traditional attitudes bind women into low paid, low status jobs and the lower grades of occupations. Whilst these may not be life-threatening, they do involve their own particular occupational health hazards. Of equal importance from a health perspective, however, is the burden created by the double day of paid and domestic labour that many women experience. In one study of women factory workers, this situation was described in the following terms:

'Women are caught in a constant and unremitting round of activity throughout their waking hours. Their work begins early, about 5 or 6 a.m. and finishes late, about 9 or 10 p.m. with little or no time for relaxation, leaving them continuously tired and often emotionally exhausted. Many are responsible for the household budget and under financial pressure to make ends meet, which is a major factor in their going out to work.'

Recently there have been important changes in the patterns of morbidity and mortality amongst women. In particular, the incidence of conditions which have traditionally been viewed as male diseases – lung cancer and heart disease, for example – are rising, whilst the incidence of psychological distress also continues to be high. From 1978 to 1984, for example, the standardized mortality ratio (SMR) for lung cancer amongst females rose from 100 to 127 during a period when the overall SMR for females fell from 100 to 92.

In seeking to explain these recent trends, some commentators have focused on a particular disease: the increasing incidence of lung cancers, for example, has been linked to changes in patterns of cigarette smoking amongst women. Others take a somewhat different perspective, concentrating not on aspects of individual behaviour, but on the social and economic changes in women's lives. According to the sociologist Lesley Doyal, for example, the increasing incidence of what she terms 'these *diseases of liberation*' reflects the fact that:

'the gains of "liberation" have in many ways been illusory – that women have gained the right to work in the world outside, but often on very unhealthy terms. That is to say, they are now exposed to new stresses and hazards outside the home, but without being relieved of their traditional role obligations and this "double burden" is reflected in their changing patterns of morbidity and mortality.'

Ethnicity, racial discrimination and health inequalities

The social and economic disadvantages experienced by black minority ethnic groups have been referred to at several points in this chapter. Black Britons are concentrated in lower social classes with limited employment opportunities, low incomes and poor housing. There are, of course, other minority ethnic groups in Britain, such as the Irish, who are also socially and economically disadvantaged and whose health is relatively poor in comparison with the white majority ethnic group.

It is important to note, however, that a large part of the explanation for the disadvantaged position of black people in Britain is the racial discrimination they experience in all walks of life. A survey of the living standards of black and white Britons conducted in 1981, for example, found that the pattern of poor jobs amongst black workers could be partly explained by poor educational qualifications, a lack of fluency in English and the different residential locations of black communities. But such individualistic and historical factors could not explain all of the disadvantage; rather, as the authors of the report concluded:

'Our expectation . . . was that we would find a substantial reduction in levels of inequality . . . instead we find a complex jumble of new inequalities, rooted in three linked problems. First, it is clear that racism and direct racial discrimination continue to have a powerful impact on the lives of black people. Second, the position of the black citizens largely remains that allocated to them as immigrant workers in the 1950s and 1960s. Third. . . the organization and institutions of British society have policies and practices that additionally disadvantage black people because they frequently take no account of the cultural differences between groups with different ethnic origins.'

Racial discrimination, then, is a major factor in generating social and economic conditions which adversely affect the health of black people in Britain directly, in terms of living standards, and indirectly in terms of the psychological impact of living in a racist society. The most obvious manifestation is racially motivated harrassment and physical attacks. In 1981, the Home Office published a report of the incidence of racially motivated offences – including all incidents, not just personal attacks – brought to the attention of the police over a three-month period. The rate per hundred thousand population was 1.4 for whites, 51.2 for West Indians and Africans, and 69.7 for Asians. The authors of the study mentioned earlier, however, suggest that the actual frequency of racial attacks could be over ten times the figure calculated by the Home Office. Whatever the actual figure, it is clear that, as the Home Office report noted, the incidence of racial attacks is a significant problem generating a great deal of anxiety and concern – not to mention physical injury – amongst black communities.

Distribution of income and health inequalities

This chapter has considered a number of different dimensions of deprivation which can be expected to contribute to the patterns of inequalities in health described in the introduction. Whilst these have been discussed as separate issues, is it important to stress that they coalesce to create a complex, health damaging environment over which individuals have little, if any, control. One way of looking at the link between health and this broader social and economic environment is to consider the relationship between the overall distribution of income in a society and the distribution of 'ill health' variously measured.

Both cross sectional and longitudinal data have suggested that the more equal the distribution of *income* in a society, the more equal the *life expectancy* of different social groups. In a recent book, Richard Wilkinson argued that across the 11 OECD (Organization for European Cooperation and Development) countries for which reliable data are available, there is a correlation coefficient of better than -0.8 between coefficients of income inequality after tax and both life expectancy and infant mortality. Wilkinson also cited the work of the social historian Jay Winters who showed that the decades 1911–21 and 1940–51 saw the most rapid improvement this century in the life expectancy of civilian men and women. He argued that these improvements were primarily due to what he refers to as 'an unanticipated but real improvement in the standard of living of the home population' during a period which, as Wilkinson has pointed out, was characterized by a narrowing of income differences.

One of the most vivid examples of the link between the distribution of income in a society and the distribution of health is provided by the small state of Kerala in South West India. Since its formation in 1956, Kerala has pursued policies of income distribution through, for example, reform of the land tenure system, employment security, free education at primary level and some redistribution of health care resources away from urban areas. With a gross national product per capita far lower than many other states, such as the Punjab and Maharashja, Kerala is relatively poor. By 1981, however, the people of Kerala had a life expectancy at birth of 63.8 years and an infant mortality rate of 39.1 per 1000 live births, compared with a life expectancy of 52 years and infant mortality of 125 per 1000 live births in India as a whole.

POLICY IMPLICATIONS OF HEALTH INEQUALITIES

In 1890, Sir John Simon – the leading health reformer of the nineteenth century – noted that:

> 'in the whole range of questions concerning the Public Health there is not, in my opinion, any one to be deemed more important . . . I doubt if any can be considered more essential or ought to be hoped

for with more ardent hope than that the poverty of our poorer classes may be lessened.'

Ninety years later, Jerry Morris, a community physician, argued in the pages of the British Medical Journal that Simon's question was no less relevant to public health. In the late twentieth century he has suggested:

'. . . we are still beset by nineteenth century type problems of deprivation. If we are to be rid of social inequalities in health these will have to be resolved at the same time as more focused education and health service measures are instituted and the initiatives provided for changes in life-styles, diet and exercise, and smoking and drinking behaviour.'

John Simon's question 'how the poor are to be made less poor' inevitably raises the question of whether and how the rich should be made less rich. Wilkinson, whose research on the relationship between the distribution of income and health was referred to earlier, also addressed this question, and estimated the advantages to be gained in health terms from pursuing a policy of greater income redistribution in the UK:

'Every pound transferred from people earning (in 1970) £60–70 per week to people earning £20–30 would reduce the death rates of recipients by five times as much as it increased those of the donors.'

The Black Report also concluded that a radical programme to improve the income and general living conditions of poorer people was essential. The report outlined a comprehensive anti-poverty programme which would not only improve national standards but also 'encourage self-dependence and a high level of individual skills and autonomy as a basis for creating a more integrated society.'

It is, however, at the clinical and personal level, in their day-to-day practice, that doctors and other health service staff can do most to help patients whose social and economic circumstances damage their health. The winds of change are undoubtedly being felt within primary care in the late 1980s. There has been a plethora of reports recently, including a White Paper published in 1987 entitled *Promoting Better Health*, the Green Paper which preceded it entitled *Primary Health Care: An Agenda for Discussion*, and the Cumberlege Report on *Community Nursing*. Some of these reports are discussed in greater detail in other contributions to this volume; they contain a number of suggestions for reorganizing care which offer the potential to develop a health service more relevant to the needs of disadvantaged people.

It is argued, but by no means generally agreed, that a more integrated service with democratically elected health authorities, for instance, could result in a more flexible service, sensitive to local needs and with a greater emphasis on prevention. Additionally, as the research of Beale and other general practitioners such as Brian Jarman has suggested, health services in areas where social and economic disadvantage is intense need more resources.

There are also practical ways in which primary health services can improve living conditions. Welfare rights services, for example, are being introduced in some health centres and surgeries, but they should and could be more widespread. In 1981, more than £900 million of benefits were unclaimed by those eligible, and primary care services are an important means of reaching these people.

A reorganized health service should also include projects based on the community development model. Community health groups have already been developed in many parts of the country, focusing on the problems of specific sectors such as black minorities. These groups also take up wider health issues – for example, poor housing, lack of play space and leisure facilities, and environmental pollution. However, they face many difficulties, in particular that of gaining the recognition and support of the health professions.

If primary health services are to make a more effective contribution to reducing health inequalities, they also need to be more aware of the nature and scale of social and economic disadvantage at both an area and an individual level. Some work is already going into developing effective ways of recording the employment status of patients for example, but medical records should include information on other social and economic factors that might adversely affect health, such as the employment history of individuals (including the chemical and physical hazards they are exposed to) or the housing circumstances of families. The privacy of patients is an important issue, so too is the way in which such information is interpreted. Lone parent status, for example, is undoubtedly an important 'risk factor', but it is not lone parenthood per se that will adversely affect health; rather, it is the poverty, housing difficulties, social isolation and other dimensions of deprivation which often accompany it.

There is also the question of how such information is to be used. At the simplest level, it can create wider awareness of the social and economic factors which strongly influence the health choices that individuals can make. As Beale's study and those of other general practitioners illustrate, however, such information can also make an important contribution to the debate about the causes of health inequalities and the implications for health services and wider social and economic policies. In the context of unemployment, Richard Smith of the British Medical Journal has argued that:

'Responding to this problem will be a challenge to the "modern general practitioner" and it is one that few have yet taken on.'

The same, with even greater emphasis, can be said for the other aspects of deprivation which underlie inequalities in health in contemporary Britain.

REFERENCES AND FURTHER READING

Brown, G., Harris T. (1978). *Social Origins of Depression: A Study of Psychiatric Disorder in Women*. London: Tavistock Publications.

Department of Health and Social Security (1986). *Low Income Families, 1983*. Unpublished Memo.

Donovan J. (1984). Ethnicity and health: a research review. *Soc. Sci. Med.*, **19**, 663.

Fagin B., Little L. (1984). *The Forsaken Families*. Harmondsworth: Penguin.

Finch J., Groves D. (1983). *A Labour of Love: Women, Work and Caring*. London: Routledge & Kegan Paul.

Graham H. (1984). *Women, Health and the Family*. Brighton: Health Education Council/Wheatsheaf Books.

Graham H. (1986). *Caring for the Family*. Health Education Council Research Report 1. London: Health Education Council.

Land H. (1977). Inequalities in large families – more of the same or different? In *Equalities and Inequalities in Family Life* (Chester R., Peel J., eds) pp. 174–5. London: Academic Press.

Lansley S., Weir S. (1983). Towards a popular view of poverty. *New Society*, 25th August, 284.

Martin R., Wallace J. (1984). *Working Women in Recession: Employment, Redundancy and Unemployment*. Oxford: Oxford University Press.

Open University (1985). Contemporary patterns of disease. In *The Health of Nations* Book III: *Health and Disease*, Chapter 9. Milton Keynes: Open University Press.

Report of a Research Working Group on Inequalities in Health (Black Report; 1980). London: HMSO.

Smith R. (1986). Improving the health of the unemployed: a job for health authorities and health workers. *Br. Med. J.*, 292, 470.

Stellman J. M. (1977). *Women's Work, Women's Health: Myths and Realities*. New York: Pantheon Books.

Townsend P. (1979). *Poverty in the United Kingdom*. Harmondsworth: Pelican Books.

Verbrugge L. M. (1985). Gender and health: an update on hypotheses and evidence. *J. Health Soc. Behav.*, 26, 156.

Wilkinson R. G. (1986). Income and mortality. In *Class and Health: Research and Longitudinal Data* (Wilkinson R. G., ed.) pp. 88–114. London: Tavistock Publications.

4

Epidemiology and Prevention in General Practice

THE PRACTICE POPULATION • CONSULTATION PATTERNS IN GENERAL PRACTICE • HEALTH FOR ALL • PREVENTION AND HEALTH PROMOTION IN GENERAL PRACTICE • CHILD CARE • THE ELDERLY • CONCLUSION

On an average working day, about 650 000 people are seen by their family doctor and at least 100 000 are visited by nurses or other health workers in the community. The number of general practitioners in the UK contracted to provide general medical services has risen by 11% from 26 345 in 1979 to 29 137 in 1984. The cost of these services in the UK (excluding the cost of medicines prescribed or hospital investigations requested by general practitioners) was about £1.2 billion in 1984–5.

Ninety-eight per cent of people are registered with a family doctor. In the decade to 1984, the average number of patients on a general practitioner's list fell by over 12% to around 2000 and a further fall is expected.

THE PRACTICE POPULATION

In order for the general practitioner and other members of the primary care team to play an effective part in prevention, it is essential for them to have adequate knowledge of the characteristics of the practice population as well as of the patients as individuals. For instance, an inner city practice population with a diversity of ethnic groups will have different needs from a dispersed rural population. An *age/sex register* which is continually kept up to date is essential to planning and monitoring in general practice. It records each patient registered within a general practice and enables systematic surveillance of various age groups to be undertaken; it is also invaluable for research. Age/sex registers may be maintained both by the practice and by the Family Practitioner Committee, which undertakes the payment of general practitioners and the administration of Family Practitioner Services. The number of patients on age/sex registers tends to be somewhat inflated because of the difficulty in keeping up with patients' movements, particularly in a mobile urban population. A few patients may actually seek to register with two practices, for instance, if they live in one area and work in another. Delays in the registration of new arrivals only partly compensate for the inflation of numbers. Temporary residents may introduce another difficulty particularly in holiday resorts where the population may increase markedly during the summer, although they would not normally be entered on the age/sex register. With the rapid computerization of Family Practitioner Committee records (virtually complete by April 1988), it is becoming increasingly easier for general practitioners to obtain accurate age/sex registers, and for Family Practitioner Committees to control inflation of list sizes.

CONSULTATION PATTERNS IN GENERAL PRACTICE

There are large differences between doctors in their patient consultation rates per day. In some cases, the reasons for consultation may be clear – an acute medical problem or follow-up of a chronic condition. In many instances, however, the understanding of consultation patterns can be approached only by taking into account several characteristics of both patient and doctor, as well as the social and family environment in which the patient lives.

Consultation may be initiated by patients (or, in the case of children, by parents), by relatives and neighbours or by the general practitioners and other members of the primary health care team. *Trigger factors* which may result in patients consulting can include physical symptoms which exceed the limits of the patient's tolerance (for example pain, dyspnoea, cough), or psychological or social stress for which a range of tolerance exists. On occasions, consultations may be deferred by the patient when there is a medical need for urgency. Conversely, patients may consult with what may appear to be trivial or 'irrelevant' symptoms. The patient and doctor may have different aims and perspectives which can lead to a discordance in how they view the consultation; for instance the doctor, in attempting to make a conventional diagnosis, may overlook the patient's real needs and concerns.

There are several *characteristics of the doctor or practice* which may affect consultation rates and patterns, including age, sex, postgraduate training, list size, practice organization, policy on repeat prescribing and attitudes to the management of chronic disease. The nature of the population (inner city, rural etc.) and the social class distribution may also be of relevance. It is well known, for example, that female patients may prefer to consult female doctors particularly for gynaecological problems and contraception. Older doctors may tend to keep with them an older list of patients. Several studies have suggested, however, that much of the variation in consultation rates cannot readily be explained by the measurable factors listed above. Consultation patterns appear to be characteristic of the individual doctor and show considerable consistency over time.

In London, inner city primary care suffers from having an excess of elderly single-handed practitioners with a relative lack of facilities and attached staff. This pattern does not necessarily apply to other inner city populations; for instance, a study of area variations in the process of care in urban general practice from Manchester did not show major differences in types of problems or the care received compared with those in outer areas of the city.

The majority of consultations occur at doctors' surgeries, but *home visiting* continues to be an important, if declining, part of a general practitioner's work in the UK (reducing from 17% of all consultations in 1971 to 12% in 1981). Most commonly, home visits are to the very young and the elderly. General practitioners can also request domiciliary visits by consultants, and these have increased almost fourfold between 1948–9 and 1979–80; more recently, however, there appears to be a decline. The specialties most frequently involved in domiciliary consultations are geriatric medicine and psychiatry. Domiciliary consultations may, on occasions, be used to expedite admission to hospital, although less than one quarter result in admissions being arranged. Unfortunately, the opportunity for joint consultation by general practitioner and hospital consultant is frequently missed – in only a minority of cases do the general practitioner and consultant see the patient together.

Accessibility of primary health care

In general in the UK, few patients experience difficulties in reaching the general practitioner's surgery. A large survey of around 5000 individuals in the UK showed that 94% found the journey fairly or very easy. However, there appear to be variations by *social class*, with 69% of people in social class I finding it very easy to get there compared with 55% of those in social class V. Predictably, *elderly* patients find it more difficult to get to their doctor, not only because of the infirmities of age but also because they are less likely to have the use of a car. About three quarters of respondents in this survey reported that their general practitioners used appointment systems, which were particularly common in larger group practices. Overall, 17% of practices were single-handed and, at the other extreme, 11% had six or more doctors.

Receptionists are employed in over 90% of practices. More than three quarters of the respondents had favourable views of the receptionist, and a similar proportion saw the receptionist as no hindrance to access to the doctor. The majority of individuals (76%) viewed their doctor as approachable and their views were to some extent related to how often they had sought their doctor's advice. Those with the most favourable view were likely to have consulted their doctor ten or more times in the previous year.

Very few people actually *change doctor* except when they are forced by circumstances to do so, but rather more people *consider* doing so. Only 2% of the study population had changed to their present doctor in the last ten years because they were dissatisfied with their former general practitioner, but 9% had actually considered doing so. Around 80% of respondents thought that it was fairly or very easy to get the doctor to make a daytime home visit. Amongst those who attempted to contact their doctor outside surgery hours, two thirds were visited by a doctor from their own practice.

Diagnostic classification in general practice consultations

The diagnosis and categorization of disease in general practice is often much less clear-cut than in hospital patients. Once a patient has reached hospital, either by referral from a general practitioner or self-referral to an accident and emergency department, considerable selection has occurred and some form of diagnostic label has frequently been applied. In general practice, many consultations conclude without a clear-cut diagnosis being made. In some cases, this is because the general practitioner is using *time* itself as a diagnostic device to separate those who have evolving symptoms from those who have self-limiting conditions. This is more acceptable in general practice than hospital medicine because many illnesses present in their early stages with non-specific symptoms and detailed investigations are unwarranted and unnecessary at this point. Review of a patient after a period of time has elapsed allows the general practitioner to assess more clearly the likely cause of the patient's symptoms and whether further investigation is necessary. Some conditions in general practice undergo changes in *diagnostic labelling* as knowledge advances. For instance, many children are treated unnecessarily with antibiotics for 'recurrent bronchitis' or recurrent coughs, but it is now clear that a considerable number of them are suffering from asthma. Increasing recognition of this by general practitioners leads to improved management but is likely to result in asthma in childhood showing a pronounced but spurious increase.

Several *classification systems* have been proposed for diagnoses in general practice. In the UK, the Royal College of General Practitioners has developed a system which is derived from and compatible with the Ninth Edition of the International Classification of Diseases of the World Health Organization. There is also an *International Classification of Health Problems in Primary Health Care* and, more recently, an *International Classification of Process in Primary Health Care* has been devised which allows classification of procedures. In 1986, James Read, a general practitioner, introduced a system of classifying diagnoses, investigations, referrals and other aspects of medical activity. This system is comprehensive and has been used in computer systems, which are rapidly gaining popularity in general practice. The use of a standard classification system permits epidemiological studies of the incidence and prevalence of conditions in general practice. Although they cannot solve all the difficulties of diagnostic categorization in primary care because of the problems of definition, the use of such a system helps to minimize diagnostic discrepancies between doctors.

Factors affecting consultation rates

The first national study of morbidity in general practice took place in 1955–6, the second in 1970–1 and the third in 1981–2. One of the purposes of these studies was to examine the relationship between *social class* and consultation rate. Amongst children aged 0–4 years, there is a tendency for the patient consultation rate (the number of children consulting per year per 1000 at risk) to peak in social class III N (non-manual), despite a tendency for the episode rate for illness to be higher amongst those of lower social class. This may be because parents in lower social classes with young children may be less likely to consult with minor illness in their children than are better-off parents. The discrepancy in patient consulting rates by social class is particularly marked for preventive procedures and medical examinations, where attendance is much lower amongst children of lower social class families. Amongst older children (aged 5–14 years), patient consulting rates tend to rise somewhat with descending social class and the gradient is particularly marked for accidents, poisoning and violence. Amongst adults aged 15–64 years, the standard patient consulting ratio (which takes into account age differences in practice populations) rises with descending social class in both cases. However, the increase is much less marked than the association between standardized mortality ratios and social class, suggesting that lower social class adults may not be consulting as much as their level of ill health suggests they should – assuming, of course, that consultations might have a beneficial effect on their state of health! Further analyses of patterns of consultations (by social class) have shown that the rate of initial consultation for an illness is very similar across social class, but rates for subsequent consultations show a steep trend from social class I to V. General practitioners may attempt to 'compensate' in some way for the relative deficit of consultations amongst patients of lower social classes by recalling them more frequently.

In general, females consult more frequently than males, the difference being particularly marked in the 15–44 year age group. It is only in children aged under five years that the consultation rate for males slightly exceeds those for females. The marked *female excess* (approximately double the male rate) amongst the 15–44 age group is partly due to visits for contraception, antenatal care and cervical smears, but these categories do not by any means explain all of the difference. Large excesses in consultation rates for women are also seen for diseases of the genito-urinary system, particularly cystitis, and of course for menstrual disorders and vaginal discharge. Large excesses for females are also particularly striking for mental disorders – specifically, both anxiety and depressive neuroses.

A comparison of data from the three *National Morbidity Surveys* mentioned above suggests a moderate rise in patient consulting rate, and a slight rise in the number of consultations per episode of illness, between the last two surveys. The rise in patient consulting rate was particularly obvious amongst the young (aged less than 14 years) and elderly (over 65), and was seen across a range of diagnostic categories. Between 1971–2 and 1981–2, referrals for both in- and outpatient care seem to fall slightly; however, interpretation was complicated somewhat by the use of slightly different categories of referral between the two surveys. Home visiting as a percentage of all consultations has also fallen. The numbers of consultations per person at risk per annum from the Third National Morbidity Study are given in Table 4.1. As one would expect, the number of consultations was highest for the 0–4 and 65–74 year age groups in both sexes. The percentage of consultations for 18 main disease classifications are shown in Table 4.2. It can be seen that respiratory conditions represent the most common reason for consultation, followed by cardiovascular conditions in men and mental disorders in women.

Table 4.1 *Consultation rates per 1000 persons at risk by age and sex (Third National Morbidity Study, 1981–2)*

	All ages	0–4	5–14	15–24	25–44	45–64	65–74	75 and over
				Age (years)				
Males	2711	5156	2040	1746	1984	3047	4103	5231
Females	4021	4659	2119	4165	4203	3928	4590	5491

Perceptions of the consultation

Studies of general practice conducted in both 1964 and 1977 by Cartwright and Anderson, suggested that over this period the views of patients and their doctors had changed comparatively little, despite a considerable increase in expenditure on general practice and the

Table 4.2 *Percentage of consultations for persons (male and female) consulting their general practitioner for 18 main disease classifications in England and Wales (Third National Morbidity Study, 1981–2)*

	Category of condition	Males %	Females %
(1)	Infections and parasitic diseases	6.0	4.9
(2)	Neoplastic diseases	1.5	1.1
(3)	Endocrine nutritional and metabolic diseases	1.9	2.4
(4)	Diseases of the blood and blood-forming organs	0.3	0.6
(5)	Mental disorders	5.3	7.7
(6)	Diseases of the nervous system and sense organs	9.0	6.8
(7)	Heart disease and hypertension, and other diseases of the circulatory system	10.3	8.0
(8)	Diseases of the respiratory system	19.8	13.7
(9)	Diseases of the digestive system	4.7	3.5
(10)	Diseases of the genito-urinary system (including breast)	2.1	6.7
(11)	Diseases of pregnancy etc.	–	0.8
(12)	Diseases of the skin and subcutaneous tissue	6.8	5.4
(13)	Arthritis, rheumatism and other diseases of the musculoskeletal system	9.1	8.2
(14) & (15)	Congenital anomalies and perinatal diseases	0.2	0.1
(16)	Symptoms and ill-defined diseases	8.3	8.1
(17)	Accidents, injury, poisoning and violence	7.2	4.3
(18)	Supplementary classification (includes prevention, family planning, administrative procedures, maternity care, social/marital problems etc.)	7.6	17.8
	Total all consultation	100.0	100.0

development of group practices, vocational training, increased ancillary staff and more cover for night calls and periods of sickness. This suggests that expectations have kept pace with improvements in medical care. There was a marked fall in doctor dissatisfaction with inadequate leisure time and rather more doctors enjoyed the diversity of their work in the later study; however, the majority felt they were more busy in 1977 than ten years previously even though this study found little change in overall consultation rates and a marked decrease in home visits. In both studies two thirds of patients came away from the surgery with a prescription; by 1977, the cost of drugs prescribed by general practitioners was about one and a half times the cost of providing the general practitioner services (and has remained at about this level).

About one quarter of general practitioners regarded at least half of their consultations as trivial, inappropriate or unnecessary in both 1964 and 1977. The general practitioners who regarded a high proportion of consultations as trivial, carried out few procedures themselves, had access to limited diagnostic tests and attended few courses. In the later survey, doctors were less likely to feel that it was appropriate for patients to consult them with problems in their family lives, but at the same time they felt there was an increasing trend for patients to seek help from them in this area. The fall in home visiting between the two studies was a frequent cause of criticism by the patients. Although some of the decline may be explained by greater car ownership, the decrease in consultations in the home may weaken the doctor-patient relationship if it results in a poorer understanding by general practitioners of their patients' home circumstances.

Psychosocial diagnoses

There is an enormous range in the diagnosis of psychiatric disorder by general pratitioners which is not explained by the variation in the psychiatric morbidity of the populations that they serve. It is likely that the *personality* and *attitudes* of the general practitioner are important determinants in the frequency with which he or she makes a psychiatric diagnosis. The pioneer work of Michael and Enid Balint, who studied the content of the general practice consultation, has shown that in some cases the doctor's attempt to make a clinical diagnosis along the lines familiar in hospital medicine may not lead to an understanding of the patient's needs. Their approach sought to help doctors to recognize and understand their patients' complaints, not only in terms of illness but also in terms of personal conflict and problems. This understanding may have a therapeutic effect if used appropriately. Experienced practitioners may often be able to tune in to patients' needs without asking large numbers of questions. This entails being aware of the reactions that patients elicit from their doctors. The emotional reactions of the doctor to the patient may be useful indicators of diagnostic importance. There seems little doubt that positive feelings of general practitioners towards their work are related to greater openness to patients and to giving more attention to psychosocial aspects of the consultation. Conversely, feelings of frustration, tension and lack of time may be associated with a high rate of prescribing and poor communication with patients.

A general practitioner with a list size of around 2500 patients would be expected to see about 100–125 new psychiatric cases a year. Many of the patients are likely to be suffering from *'neurotic depression'*: the majority of such patients are managed solely in general practice. Diagnosis by general practitioners may be inappropriate, and there has been criticism that general practitioners may miss depression or wrongly diagnose it in patients who are not depressed. Moreover, many doctors may inaccurately judge the severity of emotional disturbance. A recent study found that half of the patients with severe depression screened in the waiting room went unrecognized by their general practitioner. Physical illness was present in 30% of the unrecognized group and depression seemed related to it. The unrecognized patients were rather more likely to have had their symptoms for more than a year; they were also less likely to complain of depression or admit to feeling depressed, although standard psychiatric interviews indicated that they were indeed suffering from depression.

Several studies have suggested that *adverse life events*, such as bereavement, unexpected crises or failure to achieve various life goals, may precipitate neurotic illness, particularly in those with poor social relationships and inadequate social support.

Undetected symptoms

Population studies have indicated that large numbers of people in the community have symptoms, most of which are self-treated following advice from family or friends. Individuals are much more likely to take *physical* symptoms to a doctor than *mental* ones.

The comment is sometimes made that patients bring too many trivial symptoms to their general practitioner. Some studies have attempted to measure the balance between symptoms which cause concern to patients but are not taken to doctors and apparently trivial symptoms which lead to 'inappropriate' consultations. A study in a deprived area of Glasgow suggests that the *'iceberg'* of symptoms which caused concern to patients (as judged by grading for pain, disability, serious-ness and duration according to the patient's perception) but did not result in a consultation is considerably greater than the amount of '*trivia*', judged by the same grading, presented to general practitioners. Overall, the amount of iceberg illness was around two and a half times that of possible trivia which patients brought to doctors. Females, particularly middle-aged and elderly, were more likely than males to have iceberg symptoms. Also patients with poorer education or lower social class were more likely to have iceberg symptoms. Poor accessibi-lity and lack of a telephone may have contributed to the reluctance to attend, but the patients' beliefs about symptoms being an inevitable part of ageing, or fears about possible diagnosis, may well have played a part. Neuroticism (as measured by answers to a short series of questions) was not associated with a tendency to refer medical symptoms formally, but *was* associated with having iceberg symptoms. This study indicates that, at least in a deprived urban population, there is a considerable volume of symptomatology that is not presented to primary care services even when direct financial costs (apart from prescription charges) are absent.

In trying to understand as best possible the reasons for consultation with general practitioners, it is necessary to approach the question from several different perspectives. The formal epidemiological approach can provide a measure of understanding, as can consider-ation of psychosocial characteristics, but it is also necessary to take into account patients' own beliefs about health and illness and their expectations, both of their own level of functioning and of the role of medical services.

HEALTH FOR ALL

The Thirtieth World Health Assembly in May 1977 resolved that: 'The main social target of governments and WHO in the coming decades should be the attainment by all citizens of the world by the year 2000 of a level of health that will permit them to lead a socially and economically productive life.' In the European Region of the World Health Organization, which includes 33 active member states, targets have been established that are intended to stimulate the debate on national health policies. The aims of health improvements are fourfold:

(1) *To ensure equity in health* between and within countries, initially by reducing differences in health levels between countries and between different population groups within countries by at least 25% by the year 2000.

(2) *To add life to years* by ensuring the full development and use of physical and mental capacity to cope with life in a healthy way.

(3) *To add health to life* by increasing the number of years free from major diseases and disabilities.

(4) *To add years to life* by reducing the number of premature deaths, thus increasing life expectancy at birth in the region to at least 75 years. This includes reducing mortality from accidents by at least 25%, from diseases of the circulatory system by 15%, and from cancer by at least 15%.

The targets also include:

- The abolition of measles, polio, congenital rubella, diphtheria and congenital syphilis.
- 'Significant increases' in positive health behaviour, such as balanced nutrition, non-smoking etc. (clear targets were recommended for each state, such as a minimum of 80% of the population as non-smokers).
- Programmes aimed at reducing alcohol consumption by at least 25%.

As part of the *health for all* approach, it was suggested that each member state should develop effective mechanisms for ensuring quality of patient care and health information systems to support their national strategies. Primary health care was seen as being the basis of any health system supported, of course, by secondary and tertiary care.

Whilst the UK system of primary health care contains many of the elements mentioned in the World Health Organization European Regional publication, such as the concept of team work between health workers and economic accessibility, there are several areas where improvements are indicated. There is a lack of public participation in the UK system, although increasingly self-help groups and patient participation groups are playing an important role in lobbying for improvements in health care. Coordination between Family Practitioner Services and primary care services provided by the District Health Authority is in many cases inadequate, and quality of care initiatives are dependent on the involvement of individual practitioners with very limited capacity on the part of Family Practitioner Committees to monitor and uphold standards of care.

PREVENTION AND HEALTH PROMOTION IN GENERAL PRACTICE

The UK currently has a poor record of public health compared with other countries in Western Europe. Mortality from cardiovascular disease is high, particularly in Scotland and Northern Ireland. Mortality from cancer of the cervix has fallen very little, from 2434 deaths in 1968 to 2068 in 1980, despite a massive increase in the number of cervical smears undertaken by general practitioners. Immunization rates are lower than many other developed countries.

The defined practice population provides important opportunities for prevention. Around 70% of registered patients see their general practitioner each year, and about 90% over a three-year period. The consultation can, therefore, be used as an opportunity for *prevention*. The use of the consultation to detect preventable conditions is described as *case finding* to distinguish it from *screening* in which patients are called up specifically for the purpose of detecting conditions amenable to prevention. General practice includes examples of screening, in particular the cervical smear programme, but the majority of preventive activity is undertaken in routine consultations. In very brief consultations, preventive activities tend to be omitted. It is to be hoped that, as general practice list sizes decrease, preventive activities will take up more of the time of primary health care teams. One of the advantages of the case finding approach, in addition to the economical use of resources, is that it may be more likely to include those at high risk of conditions such as heart disease, lung cancer and cervical cancer than would a screening strategy. Response rates to screening surveys tend to be lower in lower social classes, in whom the risk tends to be higher. In the case of pregnancy, attendance at postnatal examinations and receipt of contraceptive advice appears to be inversely related to a number of 'at risk' factors, including lack of a partner, social disadvantage, smoking and alcohol consumption.

Recently, there has been increasing emphasis on the concept of *health promotion* which stresses the need for changes in life-style in order to promote health. It can be considered as the process of enabling people to increase their control over and to improve their health, emphasizing social and personal resources as well as physical capacities.

Health promotion involves more than just primary care services in its implementation, but general practice nevertheless has a key role. An early example of health promotion in general practice was the Peckham

Experiment which was mounted in London in the 1930s. Situated in a deprived urban area, it combined facilities for recreation with clinical primary care and the availability of good food from a farm on the outskirts of London. Unfortunately, this project was allowed to disappear with the development of the NHS.

It has been shown that, in general, one-to-one methods of health education tend to be more effective than mass methods. This does not of course imply that the mass media of community-oriented health education are of no importance, but successful approaches are likely to include intervention at a variety of levels.

According to surveys, patients seem to welcome the involvement of general practitioners in health promotion. There is evidence that many patients who consider themselves to have a problem in the areas of smoking, alcohol, weight and fitness have not had advice from their general practitioners and would like their general practitioner to be involved.

General practitioners can help their patients to stop *smoking* by simple advice and supporting written information. Although the success rates are relatively low, perhaps 5–10%, if general practitioners around the country routinely counselled smokers the effects nationally could be considerable; their more intensive intervention might produce considerably higher cessation rates of around 20–30%.

Currently, the effect of intervention by general practitioners on heavy drinkers is being studied. The detection of *excessive alcohol consumption* may be by a standard questionnaire, standard interview, laboratory tests such as γ-glutamyl transpeptidase and mean corpuscular volume or, of course, by clinical acumen. Laboratory tests are of limited sensitivity but may be useful for monitoring progress in those cases where the parameters are raised. Common situations in which heavy alcohol consumption should be suspected include recurrent injuries or accidents, poorly controlled hypertension, sexual problems and marital disharmony, and non-specific gastrointestinal symptoms. Most heavy drinkers are unknown to their general practitioners and unless a standard history is taken in all adult patients (which is clearly impractical), many will be missed. A most cost-effective and reasonably sensitive way of recognizing heavy drinkers is by a short questionnaire which includes other areas of health concern such as smoking, exercise and weight. An alternative is for the practice nurse to include questions on alcohol during routine 'health checks'.

The safe limits of alcohol consumption are still under debate but levels of 35 units* a week for men and 21 units a week for women may be taken as reasonable guidelines above which the general practitioner should advise reduction. The *Report on Alcohol* by The Royal College of General Practitioners (1986) suggests that below 21 units per week for men and 15 units per week for women there is a 'low risk' of harm, and that there is an increasing risk above that level. For pregnant women, abstinence or minimal consumption is recommended.

Most heavy drinkers in general practice can be counselled to reduce their consumption although those who are dependent on alcohol may need to abstain. A scheme for responding to heavy drinkers was presented in the above report.

High risk and whole population approaches

There is a debate about the prevention of *ischaemic heart disease* which centres around whether intervention should be aimed at those of high risk or at the whole population, particularly with regard to lowering serum cholesterol. Selective intervention on high risk individuals would, of course, necessitate a population screening or case finding programme which so far has not seemed justified on the grounds of expense and practicality. The availability of cheap, reproducible methods of measuring lipids in the community may change these perceptions in years to come. However, a strong argument for attempting to shift the risk profile of the whole population is that the accuracy of predicting the fate of any one patient is poor. For instance, in British middle-aged men the use of the 80th percentile of cholesterol concentration would result in the detection of only about one third of those who would subsequently develop clinical ischaemic heart disease. The US National Institutes of Health sponsored a consensus development conference which recommended intensive dietary intervention for the top quarter of the distribution of cholesterol values – with the addition of appropriate drugs for the top tenth if the response to diet was inadequate. To apply similar cut-off points to British men would include around half of all middle-aged men because of their high plasma cholesterol concentrations. There is one group, however, for

---

*One unit = 8–10 g alcohol, equivalent to half a pint of beer, one glass of wine or a single measure of spirits.

whom the high risk approach is generally accepted, i.e. it is in those with first degree relatives who developed ischaemic heart disease under the age of 55 years that the plasma cholesterol concentration should be checked.

Recently, a strategy has been proposed for identifying men in the population at high risk of heart attacks which does not involve the measurement of serum cholesterol. A risk score is calculated using cigarette smoking, mean blood pressure, recall of ischaemic heart disease or diabetes diagnosed by a doctor, history of parental death from 'heart trouble' and presence of angina on a standard question-naire. The top fifth of the score distribution identified about half of the men who subsequently developed major events of ischaemic heart disease over the next five years.

General practitioners and particularly nurses in primary care can contribute to reducing the risk profile of the population by giving appropriate dietary advice. In the USA, recommendations are for a reduction in total dietary fat from 40% to 30% of total energy, including a reduction in saturated fats to 10% of total energy. In Britain, the Department of Health has recommended less dramatic reductions in total fat and saturated fats to 35% and 15%, respectively, of total energy.

The detection of *asymptomatic hypertension* by case finding is an important task of general practice. The treatment of asymptomatic hypertension is mainly justified by the reduction it produces in the incidence of stroke, but the Medical Research Council trial of mild hypertension suggested that propranolol produced a reduction in coronary events amongst non-smokers; a similar observation has been noted for men in one other major trial.

The working party of The Royal College of General Practitioners, reporting on *Health and Prevention in Primary Care*, recommended that general practitioners measure the blood pressure of all their patients over 30 years of age. There is still evidence, however, that the detection and management of patients with hypertension in general practice is inadequate. One study, for example, showed that around 50% of patients who had consulted their general practitioner within ten years had no blood pressure recording in their notes. Of those found to be hypertensive, nearly 70% had periods of longer than 12 months when no blood pressure was recorded in the notes and in addition, for those receiving treatment, blood pressure control left something to be desired.

It has been found that only about 40% of those who initially register a raised blood pressure reading will be classified as hypertensive after three readings. However, general practitioners still tend to start treatment without taking a series of readings – nearly 50% of patients treated by the general practitioners studied were given treatment after only one raised blood pressure reading. The level of blood pressure at which pharmacological treatment should be instituted is still a matter for debate and is likely to depend on age, presence of other risk factors (including a family history of cardiovascular disease) and the wishes of the patient. Since there is no threshold in the relation between blood pressure and risk, any cut-off point is bound to be arbitrary. Lower limits may be taken for the institution of non-pharmacological treatment (including reduction of obesity and of alcohol, salt and probably dietary fat intake) than for pharmacological treatment. A reasonable cut-off point for pharmacological treatment of middle-aged patients might be a sustained diastolic pressure (phase V) of 105 mmHg and/or a systolic pressure of about 170 mmHg, assuming that there are no additional risk factors or evidence of end-organ damage – if there were, pharmacological treatment may be instituted at lower levels.

The prevalence of *secondary hypertension* in a general practice hypertensive population is likely to be low (around 10% or less). Intensive investigation for secondary hypertension should focus particularly on younger patients (aged less than 40 years) or those in whom the blood pressure is difficult to control. It seems reasonable to check routinely a mid-stream urine specimen, plasma urea and electrolytes, and to ascertain whether there is evidence of cardiomegaly or retinopathy.

Obesity

Obesity is generally recognized as a risk factor for ischaemic heart disease with the risk doubling between the bottom and top fifth of the distribution of the body mass index (BMI),* which is equivalent to a difference of about 20 kg in weight. Obesity has been divided into three grades of increasing severity. Grade I corresponds to a BMI of 25.0–29.9 with little increase in mortality over this range. Grade II obesity

* $BMI = \dfrac{[\text{weight (kg)}]}{[\text{height (m)}]^2}$

(BMI = 30.0–39.9) represents the range from clinically relatively trivial to disabling obesity. Grade III (BMI >40) results in considerable impairment of the normal activities required for employment. A recent survey in one practice showed that about 40% of male patients aged 17–70 years had Grade I obesity, and about 11% were Grade II or more. Percentages for women were approximately 30% and 15%, respectively.

Treatment of patients with Grades II and III obesity may be difficult, but the general practitioner will mainly see patients with Grade I and milder Grade II obesity. The effects of consistent dietary advice and information about other factors such as exercise given by general practitioners have not been sufficiently evaluated, but in view of the simplicity of diagnosing obesity, the offer of *counselling* and *follow-up* should be made, particularly in young and early middle-aged patients.

A recent survey showed that over 80% of patients felt general practitioners should be interested in weight problems, and around 40% thought that they had a weight problem. Of these who felt they had a weight problem, approximately 40% considered that their general practitioners had not been interested.

Cervical screening

The number of cervical smears rose from 687 000 in 1965 to 2 982 000 in 1980 and general practitioners increased their contribution by twenty-fold over this period. Why has this tremendous increase in workload not resulted in a greater decrease in deaths from cancer of the cervix? It appears that women of 35 years and under may have an increased incidence of cancer of the cervix compared with cohorts born earlier. It is possible that there may be a shorter pre-invasive period in younger women. However, the major reason for the failure of death rates to decline seems to be inadequate screening of women aged between 35 and 65 years. There is a social class gradient in the incidence of cervical cancer; a higher incidence, but lower social class women tend to have lower rates of attendance for smear tests. A high proportion of women with invasive cancer have never had a smear.

General practitioners have a responsibility to ensure that all their female patients have a smear test at least every *five years* and perhaps more frequently amongst younger women. There is no longer a national recall system and it may take ten years or so for Family

Practitioner Committees to develop their own computerized recall system. The 70% reimbursement received by general practitioners for the salaries of practice nurses and other staff allows them to employ adequate practice support at very little extra net cost. Some practices have involved nurses in running a *smear clinic* where other preventive activities, such as breast self-examinations and blood pressure measurement, take place.

Family planning and *antenatal care* are both important opportunities for prevention. In addition to the opportunity to undertake cervical smears and blood pressure recordings, and to give advice about stopping smoking, rubella antibodies can be checked if there is no history of rubella immunization. More generally, both family planning and antenatal care offer opportunities for the discussion of concerns about sexuality, childbirth and child care.

CHILD CARE

There is a lack of agreement about the content of paediatric surveillance and the ages at which it should be carried out. General practitioners, health visitors and clinical medical officers employed by District Health Authorities may all be involved in these activities. Each of the health districts in the UK seems to run its own paediatric surveillance programme.

Surveillance provides the opportunity for parents and health workers to discuss child health and development. It has three main components: *health education* and guidance about child development, *screening* for specific medical problems, and *assessment of problems* presented by the parents or other relatives. The specific screening tests for which there is general agreement include: examination for cataracts, cleft palate, cardiac disease, undescended testes and congenital dislocation of the hip at six weeks. At eight or nine months, a distraction test of hearing and a test for squint are performed, and the ability of the child to sit unaided for one minute can be observed. Subsequent examinations are usually at 18 months, $2\frac{1}{2}$–3 years and 4–$4\frac{1}{2}$ years. Growth, mobility and speech can be monitored and squints checked for. Accident prevention is an important topic for discussion with parents, including hazards in the home at younger ages and road accidents in the case of older children. Parents' observations help in the identification of problems, particularly with their children's vision and hearing. With increasing numbers of general practitioners having the motivation and training to undertake paediatric surveillance, it is to be hoped that uniform policies will be adopted in the near future.

The record of *immunization* in the UK compares poorly with many other western countries. In 1983, a report showed that 23 health districts had an up-take of pertussis vaccine of less than half, while in 1984 the national up-take was only about two thirds. A total of 94 000 cases of measles were reported in England and Wales in 1982 when in the whole of the USA, only 1697 were reported in the same year. There are now national target figures for the up-take of immunization, and immunization figures are available from every district. Progress could no doubt be increased if this country had a system similar to that in the USA where completion of primary immunization is virtually mandatory for entry into school.

Table 4.3 gives the percentage of children who completed immunization by the end of the second year after birth. The fall in pertussis immunization associated with the discussion of possible adverse effects in the media, has now reversed and nearly two thirds were immunized in 1984. The adverse publicity surrounding pertussis immunization may have also affected the up-take of tetanus, diphtheria and polio vaccine for a time, although to a smaller extent.

Table 4.3   *Immunization up-take rates: percentages of children born in 1983 and immunized by the end of 1985*

Measles	68%
Pertussis (whooping cough)	65%
Diphtheria	85%
Tetanus	85%
Polio	85%

Source: DHSS.

THE ELDERLY

The vast majority (over 95%) of elderly people live in their own homes, and it is generally agreed that they should be supported and encouraged to do so.

General practitioners are paid a higher capitation fee for elderly patients which reflects, to a certain extent, the extra workload that they produce. About one third of the needs and disabilities of the elderly are unknown to health or social services personnel. This may be because old people have poor expectations of health or because they fear being taken into residential care or hospital if they appear not to be coping. Unsolicited visits to the old person may be useful for detecting problems that would otherwise remain unknown. The general practitioner or health visitor may be involved in this activity. In the 'developed' world, the numbers of elderly are increasing, particularly those aged 75 years and over. The care of the elderly is therefore likely to require increasing resources in years to come.

The functions of primary care services in providing for the elderly can be summarized under the following objectives:

(1) To help elderly people prevent unnecessary loss of function.
(2) To help elderly people prevent and treat health problems which adversely affect quality of life in old age.
(3) To supplement care given by relatives and friends, and to prevent the breakdown of these informal caring systems.
(4) To care for the dying patient.

There is still a good deal of work to be undertaken in the area of health care for the elderly in the community but it has been estimated that to set up an *assessment programme* for the over 75s in a practice of 4000 (around 200 patients) would require some 18 hours of health visitor time per week in the first year and somewhat less, say 11 hours per week, in subsequent years. A postal screening questionnaire was found to reduce the potential workload only modestly but recent studies have suggested the possibility that the workload could be reduced to about 40% requiring follow-up without compromising the efficiency of the questionnaire. A number of attributes increase the likelihood of functional decline, such as living alone, poverty, recent bereavement, recent hospitalization, problems with mobility and mental impairment. Several multi-dimensional assessments have been developed which include measures of the activities of daily living, mental and physical health and relevant social factors. They are generally too time consuming to be used routinely but it is likely that those providing primary care will increasingly adopt such an approach, perhaps in abbreviated form.

The prevalence of *dementia* is around 5–10% in patients aged over 65 years rising to perhaps 15–20% in the very elderly (aged 80 years and over). There is some evidence that many of the demented patients are unknown to their general practitioners, but more recent studies have not suggested such an 'iceberg' of dementia in the community. Results may depend somewhat on the definition used and the presence or absence of carers who may support the patient with moderate dementia, as well as the practice policies (or lack of them) for the elderly. Future trends will probably involve the primary care team as a whole with increasing development of coordinated policies by general practitioners, health visitors, district nurses and occupational therapists. Demographic changes make this an important area for increased resources and research.

Over the past 30 years, the proportion of patients who die at home has fallen from 50% to just over 25%. In a practice with about 2000 patients, about five per year may require *terminal care* at home; most but not all suffer from cancer. Experience from domiciliary terminal care teams has suggested that complete pain relief can be obtained in 80–90% of cases,with good relief in the majority of the remainder. Results as good as this may not be obtained by most general practitioners, but increasingly, health districts are developing a more coordinated policy for continuing care in the community by establishing nursing posts with a specific responsibility for this area and by improving communication between hospices and the community services.

CONCLUSION

General practitioners have a defined population for whom they have responsibility. Increasingly, they are focusing on assessing the quality of their care and this requires basic knowledge of groups at risk and measures of effectiveness such as immunization rates, extent of blood pressure recording and cervical smears. A combination of clinical skills and an epidemiological perspective is essential if general practice is to play a central role in the maintenance and improvement of public health.

REFERENCES AND FURTHER READING

Balint E., Norell J. S., eds (1973). *Six Minutes for the Patient: Interactions in General Practice Consultations*. London: Tavistock Publications.

Cartwright A., Anderson R. (1981). *General Practice Revisited.* London: Tavistock Publications.

Department of Health and Social Security (1984). *Diet and Cardio-vascular Disease.* Report on Health and Social Subjects No. 28. London: HMSO.

Kurji K. H., Haines A. P. (1984). Detection and management of hypertension in general practices in North West London.*Br. Med. J.,* 288, 903.

Ritchie J., Jacoby A., Bone M. (1981). *Access to Primary Health Care.* Office of Population Censuses and Surveys. London: HMSO.

Royal College of General Practitioners, Office of Population Censuses and Surveys, Department of Health and Social Security (1986). *Morbidity Statistics from General Practice. Third National Study 1981–2.* London: HMSO.

Royal College of Psychiatrists (1986). *Alcohol, Our Favourite Drug.* London: Tavistock Publications.

Secretaries of State for Social Services, England, Wales, Northern Ireland and Scotland (Green Paper on Primary Health Care, Cmnd. 9771; 1986). *Primary Health Care – An Agenda for Discussion.* London: HMSO.

Secretaries of State for Social Services, England, Wales, Northern Ireland and Scotland (White Paper on Primary Health Care, Cmnd. 249; 1987). *Promoting Better Health. The Government's Programme for Improving Primary Health Care.* London: HMSO.

Wright H. R. (1978). The aetiology of the consultation – a three-fold classification. *Gen. Practice.* 28, 400.

Chapter

5

The Primary Health Care Team

HISTORY AND DEVELOPMENT • RESOURCES • PREMISES •
ATTACHED AND EMPLOYED STAFF • PRACTICE
MANAGEMENT AND FINANCE • PREVENTION • THE TEAM •
THE MANAGED PROFESSIONS • INTERNATIONAL •
CONCLUSION • CAREER CHOICE

HISTORY AND DEVELOPMENT

The historical development of general practice in the UK has been described in detail in Chapter 1, but those aspects relevant to the emergence of the primary health care team warrant brief reiteration.

General practitioners originally evolved from *apothecaries* and in particular from a group of doctors in the early nineteenth century who qualified by passing the apothecarys' examination and often also the membership examination of the Royal College of Surgeons of England. The 1858 *Medical Act* established the title *registered medical practitioner* and thus general practitioners became full members of the medical profession.

For the rest of that century, these doctors usually worked alone with conditions varying widely from those who cared for the relatively affluent to those who cared for the poor. Throughout the nineteenth century, *club practice* was important; the doctor was either employed by a society to provide general medical services for patients in return for small sums paid weekly, or was contracted to provide services by an insurance-type organization.

In 1911, the Lloyd George Act (*National Health Insurance Act*) established for working men in Britain a comprehensive service, free at the time, which included a choice of doctor. This was an important step because the so-called *panel* or list of patients was the direct forerunner of the NHS list, which was to follow when the *National Health Service Act* was implemented in July 1948, in effect extending the Lloyd George Act to the whole population. The British National Health Service was thus one of the first in the world to provide a fully comprehensive service, free at the time, to every man, woman and child in the kingdom regardless of age, sex, social class or income level. Patients had a choice of doctor: doctors had a choice of patient. Medicines and referral services to hospitals were free, including investigations and inpatient and outpatient care.

The essential feature of the payment system for practitioners at that time was the *capitation fee*. The doctor was paid not in relation to the number of items of service or frequency of contact with his patient, but by the number of patients who chose to register with him. British doctors were thus paid on the Chinese system, i.e. they were essentially paid when the patients were well and not specifically paid for care when patients were ill. At this point, the arrangements in Britain diverged considerably from those of general practice in other countries in the western world where the more common fee per item of service system continued and, indeed, has remained in the majority of countries, although often modified by various forms of reimbursement for the patient by the state. The third system, that of employing salaried doctors in primary care, has never developed in any major western country nor in the North American or Australasian continents, although it has developed in Eastern Europe.

RESOURCES

In terms of government expenditure, the NHS is always one of the top four items, along with defence, education and social security. Since health and social security are handled by one department of state, the Department of Health and Social Security is the single largest spending department in government. Over 90% of the NHS is financed by *taxation*.

In the mid-1960s, Britain spent about an average proportion of its gross national product on health in comparison with other countries in Europe, and the gross national product itself was about average for countries in Western Europe. By 1983, however spending on health care in the UK was £315 per head, with only Italy and Ireland lower among European countries. This was less than half the expenditure of countries like West Germany, Switzerland and Sweden, and less than one third of the £999 per head spent in the USA.

PREMISES

In the nineteenth century and the first half of the twentieth century, general practitioners usually worked from their *homes*. There was no primary care team as we know it today – the most common assistant the doctor had was his wife, and the only other ancillary staff encountered in any numbers were receptionists. Women doctors were rare.

At the time the NHS was introduced in 1948, single-handed general practice was predominant and purpose-built premises were still rare. *Health centres*, foreseen as early as the *Dawson Report* of 1920, had never become popular but have been built in steadily increasing numbers since 1948, until now about one quarter of general practitioners work from them. The most common arrangement for most other doctors was either the 'lock-up shop' surgery, typically in big cities, or the Victorian or Edwardian house in the provinces.

It is important to understand the way in which general practitioner premises were *financed*. Given an all-inclusive capitation fee, as introduced in 1948, the doctor was heavily penalized for having good premises, or at least premises more expensive than those of the average doctor. In the mid-1960s, there was a major reform of the general practitioner's contract called the *British Medical Association Charter* which introduced for the first time a system of reimbursing the doctor in terms of *rent* for the premises actually used for the NHS. The prices were determined by the District Valuer. Reimbursement provided the doctor with a return on investment, and the Charter signalled a rapid development in general practitioner premises which underwent substantial improvement in many parts of the country. In the south-west, about 10% of trainers' practices undergo a major improvement each year.

General practitioners who practise in *health centres* do not have to provide capital for the purchase of their premises because these belong to District Health Authorities. There is, therefore, no need for capital for premises to be involved when the general practitioner joins a health centre partnership. Doctors becoming partners in partnerships which *own their building*, however, are expected to purchase a share of the premises, usually a share in proportion to the income that they will receive from the practice. This often involves younger doctors borrowing sums of money which, in effect, they are investing in the practice. Subsequently, they will receive a share of the income generated by the practice premises and returned to the partnership in the form of payments from the NHS as rent for the property. Finally, on retiring from the practice, the doctor will sell his or her share and receive a capital sum which can be particularly valuable at such a time.

ATTACHED AND EMPLOYED STAFF

One of the main pressures towards improving and developing practice premises was the need to bring more people to work together in the *primary health care team*. The definition of this team has been the subject of considerable discussion. The *core team*, which is based in one building, is currently generally accepted to include doctors, practice nurses, attached health visitors, community nurses, practice administrators, receptionists and secretaries. In some practices, midwives and other attached colleagues may form members of the core team and work from the building. In other practices, community nurses and health visitors may work mainly outside the practice.

Other members of the primary health care team, not usually based in the practice premises, include midwives, community psychiatric nurses, counsellors and dieticians. In some cases, physiotherapists and occupational therapists have been attached to practices. General practitioners increasingly work in partnership and often employ many of the core team themselves, especially their administrators, secretaries, receptionists and practice nurses. Doctors working in health centres usually have the employment arrangements made by the local health authority. Social workers in some cities and in rural areas may work from group practice centres or, more commonly, health centres, but in most parts of the country remain based in either local social services departments, which are part of local government, or as medical social workers within the hospital system.

PRACTICE MANAGEMENT AND FINANCE

The general practitioner's pay and expenses are extremely complicated and it is difficult to unravel all the arrangements. Full details are set out in the *Statement of Fees and Allowances for General Medical Practitioners* published by the DHSS and sent to every general practitioner in Britain.

The first element of finance in the doctor's pay is still the *capitation fee* which nowadays is provided at different levels according to the age of the patient, being rather more for those aged between 65 and 74 years and higher still for those aged over 75 years.

The second element of pay consists of various *allowances*, the most important of which is the Basic Practice Allowance paid to all doctors accepted by Family Practitioner Committees as principals on an NHS list, provided that they meet certain conditions, notably having over one thousand patients registered with them.

Thirdly, there are a number of *items of service* which are payable to general practitioners carrying out certain activities which are defined by the Government and agreed by the profession as desirable. These fall into two groups – those providing some particular service, notably night visits (between 11 p.m. and 7 a.m.), and those providing clinical activities mainly in the preventive field, which include immunizations and cervical smears for women in certain age groups. Special provisions are available for contraceptive care and maternity care, both of which are technically under a separate contract from general medical services in the NHS. The effect is to give general practitioners an additional fee for each patient for whom they provide contraceptive care for a year, and a set of item of service fees for those undertaking obstetric care based on the number of antenatal attendances, postnatal attendances and care in labour itself.

All these payments give an average *net NHS remuneration* for general practitioners in the UK of £26 840 in 1987–8 (non-NHS incomes are small). Younger practitioners can expect to earn less and some practitioners will obviously earn more. This average target net income is determined by the *Review Body of Doctors' and Dentists' Remuneration* which publishes an annual recommendation to the Government in April or May of each year.

A second aspect of the doctor's gross remuneration concerns *expenses* incurred in professional practice. The doctor obviously must finance the premises, including repairs, and pay for telephones, stationery, postage, heating and lighting and for certain members of the staff such as cleaners. These expenses come to about £12 500 per year (1987–8) and an average figure is allowed for them in the capitation fees and allowances provided by the Government. The effect is that if a general practitioner incurs expenses greater than the average, he or she will be financially penalized as a result.

Finally, there are a further set of *reimbursements* available to general practitioners for specific services such as premises, as mentioned above, or certain forms of ancillary staff such as receptionists, secretaries, practice administrators and practice nurses. In this case, the NHS will meet 70% of the salaries plus the National Insurance costs of these staff, as it is government and professional policy to encourage the development of the primary health care team. The doctor must pay the remaining 30% which acts as a brake on the numbers employed in this way. In fact, the average number of all ancillary staff reimbursed under this ancillary staff scheme amounts to about one whole-time equivalent staff member per general practitioner (although up to two are allowed). These direct reimbursements amount on average to about another £11 000 per general practitioner.

Taking net NHS renumeration and expenses together it means that the average general practitioner will receive about £39 000 in 1987–8 which is the so called *gross* income. It is especially important to distinguish between gross and *net* remuneration because misunderstandings about how much general practitioners earn are widespread and there is often confusion between gross income and the net amount of £26 840 that the doctor actually retains after professional expenses have been met. Given the fact that the average general practitioner has about 2000 patients, it follows that the average cost to the NHS of providing for general practitioner care for one year for the average patient is about £25 (excluding the cost of drugs prescribed and hospital investigations).

PREVENTION

In 1978, an important declaration by the World Health Organization suggested that primary health care was becoming the most important aspect of care in all health services in all countries of the world. This declaration is most usually known as the *Alma-Ata Declaration.*

General medical practice is primary *medical* care, and is an important part of primary *health* care, but the two are not the same. This is partly because of the special importance of prevention, and the World Health Organization believes that the logical method of providing frontline care in a national health service is through a multidisciplinary team which is concentrating particularly on *health promotion* and *disease prevention.* The British Government signed this declaration after it was published and is now committed to it.

THE TEAM

Teamwork is a relatively new feature of British general practice but it is growing and spreading rapidly. General practitioners remain the largest single group in the team: there are about the same number of general practitioner principals (the highest grade of general practitioner in the British National Health Service) as health visitors, community nurses and practice nurses combined.

Teamwork is becoming increasingly important to patients because it enables them to call on a wider *range of skills* than any one individual may have. Teamwork also provides the team with an opportunity to support itself by discussing difficult problems and personalities and by *sharing* the burden of responsibility and care. The acquisition of special skills is encouraged and the cost of expensive equipment, particularly computers and electrocardiograms, can be shared. Teamwork also provides for *continuity* of care and service during holidays, study leave or sickness, and provides a measure of flexibility in the organization of care.

The disadvantages of teamwork

The disadvantages of teamwork lie in problems of communication and either competition or duplication of services by different members of the team. These three problems are much more common than had been generally realized, and teamwork in primary care now requires special study to overcome them.

Communication problems can easily occur when busy individuals forget to inform each other of some new development in the patient's care and it is surprisingly easy for people to feel missed out in this way.

Competition can occur when two or more professions genuinely believe that the problem is appropriate for them and lies within their own field of activity. In fact, there is considerable overlap in the fields of activity of nurses, doctors, health visitors and sometimes midwives. Hence, there is a need for considerable discussion and definition of terms and policies if competitive care is to be avoided.

Duplication of care is sometimes deliberate policy, such as in midwifery, where women see both midwives and general practitioners simultaneously and there are transitional periods of overlap when midwives hand over to health visitors. Likewise, much child development is now shared between health visitors, practice nurses and general practitioners. Duplication is, however, potentially dangerous and expensive, and if members of different professions give different advice it can be confusing and occasionally catastrophic for patients.

Training

Few of the members of primary health care teams have received any real training in multidisciplinary work. Most have been trained separately and are then brought together; it is therefore not surprising that teams sometimes fail to generate the effectiveness and efficiency to which they aspire. One of the growing themes in primary care is *teamwork* and it is likely that this will be systematically studied and opportunities made for professions to meet and work together more in the future.

No discussion of teamwork in primary health care is complete without the stipulation that the team should meet regularly. There are certain ground rules and recipes for improving or hindering communication and all those working in primary teams today must have some understanding of *small group theory* and interaction.

Confidentiality

One of the problems often raised about teamwork in primary care is that of confidentiality. In practice, this is not such a big problem as it seems but nevertheless every member of the primary team needs to understand the principles which operate.

The first guideline is that information obtained about patients during the course of work in the practice is confidential and may not be divulged to anyone outside the practice. The second is that individuals must respect the wish of patients that certain information should be kept confidential to them alone, and this should operate equally for health visitors, nurses or doctors.

The social workers' code is slightly different and needs to be discussed and clarified within each team, if only because separate records are maintained outside the practice in a department of local government and may be accessible to other people there.

Record keeping

Another problem concerns the question of record keeping in general practice, both in terms of *access* and *availability*. Members of different professions traditionally keep separate records within the practice but the tendency to maintain a shared record is growing. Access to records needs to be clarified and practitioners should always be sure exactly who is entitled to read what.

Computers

A computer offers new methods of organizing information and in particular of recalling it rapidly. This can be especially important in many preventive programmes such as offering immunizations to children or cervical smears to women between defined ages. The computer can also provide ways of maintaining confidentiality such that only specified people can obtain access to particular sections of the computerized record.

THE MANAGED PROFESSIONS

General practitioners are *independent contractors*, that is to say they are self-employed in law and are directly accountable to their patients. They work in relation to health service authorities called Family Practitioner Committees with whom they are under contract to provide a range of services. Some of the other members of the primary care team, however, are full-time employees of local District Health Authorities. Health visitors and community nurses are in the so-called *managed* professions, that is to say their roles and responsibilities are organized or managed for them by direct superiors in a hierarchical line of accountability. In other words, there are senior health visitors or nurses, usually called *nursing officers*, to whom the practising health visitors and nurses are responsible. These officers manage staff and try to deploy them to the greatest possible advantage.

There is a potential, and sometimes real, conflict between the views of nursing officers who may be based outside the team and those of the members of the primary care team itself. A paper by Brian Jarman and Julia Cumberlege published in the *British Medical Journal* in April 1987 has suggested that much of this potential conflict can be resolved if general practitioners agree to accept patients onto their lists from defined areas which roughly overlap with the *neighbourhood nursing patches*. The team is then able to concentrate its efforts on dealing with the patients registered with the general practitioners. There is flexibility for nurses to cross the boundaries of neighbourhood nursing patches in cases where the nursing workload is not great. The few patients with greater nursing dependency who live further away can be dealt with by contacting other neighbourhood nursing managers.

INTERNATIONAL

It has been suggested that the NHS is one of the most cost-effective forms of care in the whole of the western world, and general practice is one of the most cost-effective parts of it. Although the Family Practitioner Services as a whole, that is opticians, dentists, doctors, pharmacists and the drugs prescribed, account for about one quarter of the cost of the British National Health Service, general practitioners and their expenses form only 7% of that total.

CONCLUSION

Primary care needs to be considered in relation to *secondary* and *tertiary* care. It is easy for those who have trained for many years in hospitals, whether district hospitals (secondary care) or regional or national hospitals (tertiary care), to lose their sense of proportion.

Most people get most of their care for most of the time from primary medical care services. The Government's recent discussion document *Primary Health Care – An Agenda for Discussion* states that 90% of all contacts between patients and doctors take place in general practice. The *General Household Survey* published by the Office of Population Censuses and Surveys in 1986, shows that the average patient sees his or her general practitioner about four times a year. Of even greater importance is the fact that patients in vulnerable age groups, particularly the very young and very old, consult more frequently; thus, children in the first year of life see their doctor on average six times a year, and one very important statistic from the survey is that one third of all the elderly have seen a general practitioner within the previous month. This is far more than the contact rate of any other group, including district nurses and health visitors combined.

Given that the general practitioner remains for a relatively long period in a local community, and that the average NHS patient remains registered with his or her general practitioner for about ten years (30% are registered for as long as 15 years), it follows that patients still have a good chance to develop personal relationships with general practitioners over a considerable length of time. Cartwright and Anderson reported in 1981 that as many as 55% of patients felt that their family doctor was 'something of a personal friend.'

Most of the problems brought by patients to the NHS are handled within primary health care and only between 5 and 10% are referred to hospitals. This is because general practitioners work closely with practice nurses, health visitors and community nurses, and are thus well placed to understand the full range of patients' needs. In any given 12-month period, two thirds of the British population consult a general practitioner and over 90% are seen in any five-year period. This means that planned preventive care on an opportunistic basis is certainly possible, although it does call for a very high degree of self-discipline and well organized medical records if it is to be effective.

Apart from the care of illness implicit in these figures, general practice is increasingly adopting a preventive orientation to health care. Over 90% of mothers see general practitioners for antenatal and postnatal care although most deliveries nowadays take place in hospital. Once the baby goes home, it is visited by a health visitor, and increasing numbers of general practitioners are becoming involved in planned preventive care in childhood.

The content of general practice care is changing. Much preventive advice can be very effectively given during the course of ordinary day-to-day consultations. Russell et al. (1979), for example, showed that as many as 5% of patients in London would stop smoking for at least a year if given simple advice by a general practitioner accompanied by a leaflet. Other and later studies have shown that higher percentages can be achieved by general practitioners in various circumstances. Similarly, general practice is now the place where most preventive care is given including, for example, blood pressure checks, contraceptive care and cervical smears. Some health districts have now achieved immunization rates of around 95% and most of these immunizations have been done in general practice.

All this preventive activity can be categorized under the general heading of *health promotion*. The other broad category looming consistently larger in general practice is *chronic disease*. It is clear that there are a small number of diseases that are relatively common in the population, notably asthma, diabetes, epilepsy, rheumatoid arthritis, osteo-arthritis, cardiac failure, depression and schizophrenia, where a general practitioner can make a substantial difference to the quality of patients' lives and may well be effective in increasing life expectancy. This has led to considerable interest in protocols or standards of care defined by general practitioners, which can be seen as an important trend for the future.

CAREER CHOICE

There have been important changes in the preference of British medical students in the last few years which have been particularly associated with the introduction of more teaching by departments of general practice in medical schools and the introduction of mandatory vocational training for general practice which came into force in 1981.

The latest figures show that general practice is by far the largest career choice for British medical students, and it is likely that the great scope and attractions of this kind of medicine are at last becoming more widely recognized.

REFERENCES AND FURTHER READING

Department of Health and Social Security (1986). *Statement of Fees and Allowances for General Medical Practitioners in England.* London: DHSS.

General Medical Services Committee of the British Medical Association and the Royal College of General Practitioners (1984). *Handbook of Preventive Care for Pre-School Children.* London: GMSC and RCGP.

Jarman B., Cumberlege J. (1987). Developing primary health care. *Br. Med. J.*, **294**, 1005.

Parkhouse J., Campbell M. G., Parkhouse H. F. (1983). Career preferences of doctors qualifying in 1974–1980: a comparison of preregistration findings. *Health Trends*, **15**, 28.

Report on the Future Provision of Medical and Allied Services. Interim

Report to the Ministry of Health (Dawson Report; 1920). London: HMSO.

Royal College of General Practitioners (1978). The care of children. *J. Royal Coll. Gen. Practit.*, **28**, 553.

Secretaries of State for Social Services, England, Wales, Northern Ireland and Scotland (Cmnd. 9771; 1986). *Primary Health Care – An Agenda for Discussion.* London: HMSO.

Chapter

6

Primary Care in Inner Cities

IDENTIFYING INNER CITY AREAS ● SOCIAL FACTORS,
HEALTH AND HEALTH SERVICES ● CHARACTERISTICS OF
INNER CITY PRIMARY CARE SERVICES ● THE 1987
GOVERNMENT WHITE PAPER

The reason for distinguishing inner city areas from the point of view of primary care is because there are, generally speaking, more social and medical problems in these areas which put greater demands on the primary care workers. Until the last few years, this had not been clearly recognized, and at the moment no significant allowance is made for this in the arrangements for providing general practitioner services. However, the 1981 Acheson Report on primary health care in Inner London, the 1987 Government White Paper for improving primary health care, and the Green Paper which preceded it, have all covered the topic in detail and recommendations have been made in the White Paper which could, for the first time, modify the terms of service for general practitioners in order to improve services in inner city areas – by means of a *Deprived Areas Allowance* and other changes.

A paper by Valerie Imber on *A Classification of the English Personal Social Service Authorities* published by the DHSS in 1977 suggested that social circumstances in inner cities are related to 'the exodus of the socially successful leaving behind the elderly and mothers on their own in poor housing. With the subsequent influx of those born in the New Commonwealth or Ireland . . . the inner city areas tend to contain more people who do not fit the usual pattern of society (where families usually have two parents and the elderly are cared for by their children) and immigrants are often culturally distinctive and contain a higher proportion of people whose wider family background has been disrupted. Not surprisingly, the numbers of homeless and rootless, drug addicts, alcoholics etc. is also at its highest in these inner areas, and the inner London boroughs are extreme types of inner city areas.'

The term *inner city* and its associated *deprivation* conjures up a variety of images of social, economic and health deficiencies. Typically, inner city areas are characterized by their declining manufacturing bases, falling populations, high concentrations of elderly people living alone, a high percentage of single parent families, overcrowded households, ethnic minorities, unemployment and a variety of other factors which are listed in the Acheson Report and the report of the Royal College of General Practitioners on primary care in London (Occasional Paper 16). These factors have a significant effect on mortality and morbidity patterns and also increase the pressure on the services of general practitioners and community nurses. Table 6.1 shows the average values of many of the key variables for the district health authorities of Inner London (13 districts), Outer London (18 districts) and all England (192 health districts) for 1983. To summarize briefly, almost all of the social and health status factors are worse in Inner London (the largest inner city area in the country) but the general practice factors are not adapted to deal with these conditions – there are more single-handed and elderly general practitioners and fewer primary care teams. Perhaps to compensate for these social, medical and general practice factors, there is a higher usage of hospital resources. As a consequence, hospital revenue resource reductions are planned for the period up to 1994, thus adding financial strains to the other problems which these districts face.

IDENTIFYING INNER CITY AREAS

If we wish to improve services in inner cities we must have a way of identifying the underprivileged areas we are talking about. The method has to be one which is equally applicable to all areas of the country, which can be applied to large and small areas, and which is generally accepted as fair and appropriate, particularly by those it will affect and by those who will implement it. For general practitioners, the first approach to this task is to consider where there are higher levels of

Table 6.1 *Key data – averages for district health authorities 1983 data (except social data for 1981)*

	District averages		
	Inner London	*Outer London*	*All England*
Demographic data			
Population, OPCS population			
projections, 1983	172454	262322	2 243989
% in 0–30 year age group, 1983	43.47	41.58	42.69
% in 30–65 year age group, 1983	41.31	43.21	42.22
% in 65+ year age group, 1983	15.22	15.21	15.09
Population density, persons/hectare,			
1983	85.30	38.32	17.17
Social data from 1981 census (mostly as % population)			
UPA score, eight variables	34.83	−2.02	0.00
Overcrowding	6.98	4.43	3.44
Single parent families	7.84	5.41	5.28
Women not unemployed aged 15–59,			
% economically active	90.70	94.08	92.55
Unemployed males aged 15–59,			
% economically active	14.41	8.31	11.25
Unemployed males aged 16–24,			
% economically active	17.54	11.53	15.47
All unemployed, % economically active	11.79	7.13	9.54
Under five years, % 1981	5.60	5.92	6.06
Over 65 years, % 1981	15.23	14.70	14.67
Old alone, as % over 65 years	44.87	34.50	36.27
Elderly alone, as % total population	6.87	5.07	5.32
Married	39.82	48.38	49.44
Households lacking basic amenities	10.47	5.70	4.62
Social Class V (= SEG II)	6.61	3.61	4.51
Households without a car	59.68	36.94	38.79
New Commonwealth and Pakistan	16.45	13.64	4.88
Born outside the UK	25.00	16.02	7.32
Moved house within a year	13.91	9.29	9.69
Household not owner occupier	75.20	38.87	42.98
Not in education at age 17 years	58.80	56.84	63.16
Townsend Health Index (poor health)	2.01	−1.11	0.00
Townsend Deprivation Index	7.03	−0.57	0.00
NE/NW Thames Regional Deprivation			
Index	1.06	1.01	1.03
Permanently sick, as % economically			
active	2.92	2.38	3.27
Temporarily sick, as % economically			
active	1.20	0.78	0.91

Table 6.1   *continued*

	District averages		
	Inner London	*Outer London*	*All England*
Health data			
Infant mortality rate	10.95	8.48	9.92
Perinatal mortality rate	10.33	8.72	10.30
% births less than 2500 g	8.43	7.46	6.96
SMR full age range	100	92	100
SMR to age 75 years	107	92	100
SMR to age 65 years	112	89	99
Expected deaths under 75 years, calculated from age/sex	950	1462	1356
Expected deaths, total, calculated from age/sex	2039	3101	2844
Actual deaths under age 75 years	1015	1340	1341
Actual deaths, total	2055	2874	2826
% of children born 1982 and immunized by end 1984 against			
Measles	49	59	65
Diphtheria	71	85	85
Pertussis	56	67	66
Tetanus	71	85	86
Polio	70	84	85
Primary care data			
% single-handed general practitioners	29.92	21.09	12.72
% general practitioners aged 65 years or more	15.93	9.86	5.36
Average general practitioner list size	2068	2166	2120
Community health service expenditure/1000 population, £	29175	19134	17480
Secondary care data (for all specialties except maternity and psychiatry)			
Consultants (whole time equivalents)	112.10	59.36	62.28
Consultants/100 000 population	70.39	23.07	27.00
Consultants/100 beds	9.07	6.33	6.03
Consultants + juniors/100 beds	24.12	16.92	15.75
Junior doctors (whole time equivalents)	182.100	100.100	101.100
Juniors per consultant	1.69	1.70	1.63
Beds available, all specialties except maternity and psychiatry	1243	990	1017
Beds/1000 resident population	7.61	3.79	4.33
Bed availability score (= beds/1000 with 3 × weighting for central district)	6.95	4.15	4.27

Table 6.1 *continued*

	District averages		
	Inner London	*Outer London*	*All England*
Unused beds (available-occupied/ 1000 with 4 weighting)	1.24	0.72	0.91
Expected D&Ds based on age/sex and national rates	18366	27930	25824
Actual D&Ds of resident population – except maternity and psychiatry	22088	28998	25470
Standardized D&D ratio (= actual/ expected D&Ds × 100)	120	104	100
Expected average beds used daily	566.74	859	788.35
Actual average beds used daily	727.77	925	796.48
Standardized average beds used daily, ratio	130	109	103
Expected average beds used daily rate/ 1000 resident population	3.29	3.28	3.23
Actual average beds used daily rate/ 1000 resident population	4.27	3.54	3.30
Expected LOS based on age/sex and national rates	11.3	11.2	11.1
Actual length of stay, days (LOS)	12.3	11.6	11.4
Standardized LOS (= actual/ expected LOS × 100)	109	104	103
Numbers of private nursing home beds	28	68	64
Numbers of nursing home beds	229	231	263
Nursing home beds/100 000 population	157.46	84.8	112.57
Elderly nursing home beds/100 000 population	305.30	322.6	441.15
Hospital revenue resource allocation changes (%)			
% RAWP change, regional strategic plans, 1983–4 to 1993–4	−18.19	−4.05	7.34

Note: The Inner London districts are Paddington and North Kensington, Riverside (Hammersmith and Fulham + Victoria), Tower Hamlets, City and Hackney, Hampstead, Islington, Bloomsbury, Camberwell, Lewisham and North Southwark, West Lambeth, Greenwich, Wandsworth. Some definitions of Inner London exclude Greenwich and include Newham which is, generally speaking, a more deprived district.

D&D = deaths and discharges; LOS = length of stay; OPCS = Office of Population Censuses and Surveys; RAWP = Resource Allocation Working Party; SEG = socio-economic group; SMR = standardized mortality ratio.

illness and, one might think, higher *consultation rates*. However, there
is evidence that general practitioner consultation rates do not increase
in proportion to the difficulties found in inner city areas, and that
where general practitioners are under stress patients make use of other
services, such as hospital inpatient and outpatient services which are
often more readily available in inner city areas (but more costly than
general practitioner services). Hence, it is inappropriate to measure
consultation rates alone as an indication of extra workload associated
with 'inner cityness'.

Levels of *morbidity* are also difficult to measure systematically.
Sickness claims, notification of infectious diseases, cancer registrations
and so on, have been suggested as sources of routinely collected data
which could be used to measure morbidity. However, sickness claims
are related to economic activity and apply only to the working
population, cancer registrations cover only a narrow range of morbidity, and disease notifications are incomplete and inaccurate. Hence
all are ill-suited as morbidity measures, especially in relation to general
practice. The proportion of low birth weight babies is a routinely
collected statistic which probably gives a good idea of the level of
health of the population, but it is not clear that it has direct relevance to
much of general practitioners' work.

Mortality statistics are accurately collected because of the legal
requirement for death registration, and this information can be linked
to social class because occupation is also recorded when the death is
registered. Mortality rates are best expressed as standardized values
after adjusting for the age and sex structure of the population
concerned. The number of deaths expected is calculated by applying
the national age/sex-related death rates to the age/sex structure of the
study population. The ratio of the actual to the expected deaths in a
year ($\times$ 100) is the standardized mortality ratio (SMR). Early deaths
are better indicators of ill health in an area, and so SMRs to age 75 or
age 65 years, rather than the full age range SMRs, are often used as a
health index. However, an average general practitioner will have 25
deaths per year in a list of 2000 patients and it is unreasonable to use
these as a measure of the workload associated with the 8000 consultations which a general practitioner has on average per year.

In the evidence to the Acheson Committee it became clear that
although there is a wide range of social and medical factors which
increase the stress for primary care workers, certain factors were
repeatedly mentioned and these were overwhelmingly concerned with

social rather than medical conditions. It was decided to try to develop a composite index based on social conditions which could be used as a measure of the factors that general practitioners nationally consider important in increasing their workload or pressure on their services. A questionnaire was sent to one in every ten general practitioners in the UK asking them to score, on a scale from 0 to 9, the factors which they considered increased their workload or pressure on their services when present in their area. There was a 77% response to the survey and a remarkable degree of agreement about the factors which should be considered and their relative importance.

The average weighting given to each variable by the doctors in the 115 Family Practitioner Committee areas in the UK was calculated. They differed little between the areas – for the elderly living alone the average score was 6.62 ± 0.06 (95% confidence interval). An *under-privileged area (UPA) score* was constructed based on the level of each variable in each area weighted according to the weighting from the national general practitioner survey. Before weighting, the variables were normalized with an ARCSIN (square root of the variable) transformation to make the distributions more normal, and then standardized by subtracting the mean and dividing by the standard deviation of the normalized values of all the areas being considered throughout the country. The sum of the weighted, standardized, normalized values of the variables for an area gave the UPA score. Because the values are standardized, the average value of the UPA scores for the whole country is 0 and it is found that the standard deviation is ± 16, the high scores being in areas with the worst social conditions. The weightings for the eight variables used in the score are shown in Table 6.2.

As an example, the calculation of the UPA score of Golborne Ward in the Royal Borough of Kensington and Chelsea (in the area of Portabello Road market) is shown in Table 6.3 and illustrated in Figure 6.1. The UPA score of this ward is 52.87, putting it in the top 1% of ward scores in the country. It can be seen from Table 6.3 and Figure 6.1 that this ward, in a borough which has many areas of considerable affluence, is higher than the national average particularly in terms of overcrowding and single parent households, ethnic groups, children aged under five years, unemployment and unskilled workers. All of these factors are considered by general practitioners nationally to increase their workload and pressure on their services when present in their areas. The comparison between the actual proportions of each

Table 6.2 *Variables used for UPA score – weightings and national averages*

Variable	Weighting (w)	E&W Average value	E&W normalized values Average (av)	E&W normalized values Standard deviation (sd)
Elderly living alone	6.62	5.20%	0.22574	0.04573
Children aged under five years	4.62	5.88%	0.24294	0.03198
Unskilled (SEG II, social class V)	3.74	1.83%	0.13069	0.03708
Unemployed (as % economically active)	3.34	3.20%	0.18083	0.08911
Single parent families	3.01	4.76%	0.28761	0.07834
Overcrowded (>1 person/room)	2.88	4.29%	0.23095	0.08094
Mobility (changing house in a year)	2.68	3.71%	0.30672	0.05672
Ethnic (New Commonwealth and Pakistan)	2.50	6.30%	0.12967	0.11561

E&W = England and Wales; SEG = socio-economic group.

variable and the weighted, standardized, normalized values (the components which go to make up the UPA score) shows how the importance attached to the individual variables is taken into account.

In order to evaluate the appropriateness of the UPA score, electoral ward maps were sent to five Local Medical Committees, selected to cover rural and urban areas throughout the country, who were asked to shade the maps according to their estimates of the workload or pressure on their services produced by the populations of the different wards. There was very little difference between the shading of the Local Medical Committees and the shading suggested by the UPA scores (1.2% of wards differed where complete wards were shaded, and 6.3% differed overall).

The Underprivileged Areas Subcommittee of the General Medical Services Committee of the British Medical Association, and the annual conference of Local Medical Committees have accepted the UPA score as a means of identifying deprived areas.

Professor Peter Townsend also has developed a *deprivation index* which is the sum of the standardized values of the percentages of households without cars, households not owner occupied, overcrowding and unemployment – the latter two factors being normalized with a ln (variable as a decimal + 1) transformation. Both the Townsend and

Table 6.3 *Calculation of the UPA score for the Golborne Ward*

Golborne Ward	% v × 100	%/100 v	√v	ARCSIN (√v)	Standardized[1] value	Weighted standardized[2] value
Elderly living alone	5.17	0.0517	0.227	0.229	0.080	0.527
Under-fives	8.30	0.0830	0.288	0.292	1.541	7.152
One parent families	6.02	0.0602	0.245	0.248	3.161	9.514
Unskilled	10.13	0.1013	0.318	0.324	1.606	6.005
Unemployed	18.80	0.1880	0.434	0.448	2.053	6.859
Overcrowded	24.98	0.2498	0.500	0.523	3.613	10.405
Moved house	14.62	0.1462	0.382	0.392	1.510	4.046
Ethnic	24.37	0.2437	0.494	0.516	3.344	8.361

UPA score = sum of weighted standardized values = 52.868

Notes: [1] = (ARCSIN $(\sqrt{v})$ − av)/sd
[2] = [(ARCSIN $(\sqrt{v})$ − av)/sd] × w
av = average of normalized values; sd = standard deviation of normalized values;
v = value of variable as a decimal; w = weighting.

the UPA indices are based on data from the 1981 census. These two indices give similar rankings when calculated for the District Health Authorities of England, and the correlation coefficient between them is 0.91. The 20 top scoring district health authorities on the two indices have 18 districts in common, as shown in Table 6.4. Generally speaking, the Inner London districts and other inner city areas come at the top of the list and the home counties at the bottom. Twelve Inner London districts are in the top 20 of both indices, and the top three districts in the Townsend index are all in Inner London.

The UPA scoring method, because it is based on census data, can be applied easily to *all areas* in the country, regardless of size. These range from enumeration districts (the areas covered by an enumerator at the time of the census, covering about 150 families) to electoral wards (of which there are about 10 000 in England and Wales each with an average population of about 5000), to District Health Authorities (250 000 people on average)and local authority areas. Not all areas identified by this method are in inner cities. For instance, the 100 local authority districts with the highest UPA scores (the top quarter out of a total of 403) include ten from Wales (Arfon, Ynys Mon, Merthyr

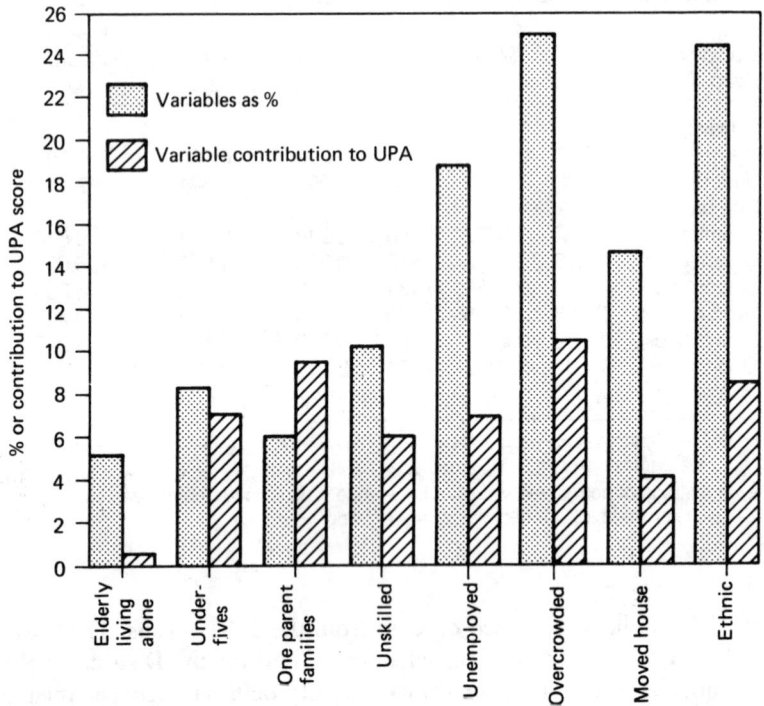

Figure 6.1 Calculation of the UPA score for the Golborne Ward. UPA score = sum of contributions = 52.87.

Tydfil, Blaenau Gwent, Cardiff, Newport, Rhuddlan, Afan, Rhymney Valley and Delyn).

The individual electoral wards with the highest scores are shown in Table 6.5. In London there is a larger geographical area of deprivation than anywhere else in the country and therefore there is a high proportion of districts in the top 20 UPA scores. However, when individual wards are studied, only three of the top 20 are in London, the highest numbers coming from Birmingham. Most of the highest scoring wards are in the North and Midlands of England. The highest in the South, outside London, is St Paul's ward in Bristol which is 36th and has a UPA score of 55.62. In Scotland, Clydeside has UPA scores

Table 6.4 *Districts with top UPA and Townsend deprivation scores*

	UPA	Townsend
1	Tower Hamlets	Tower Hamlets
2	Central Manchester	City and Hackney
3	City and Hackney	Paddington and North Kensington
4	Paddington and North Kensington	Central Manchester
5	West Birmingham	Islington
6	Camberwell	North Manchester
7	West Lambeth	West Lambeth
8	Islington	Bloomsbury
9	Bloomsbury	Liverpool
10	Bradford	West Birmingham
11	North Manchester	Camberwell
12	Newham	Hammersmith and Fulham
13	Central Birmingham	South Tyneside
14	Hammersmith and Fulham	Newham
15	Wandsworth	Lewisham and North Southwark
16	Lewisham and North Southwark	Hampstead
17	East Birmingham	East Birmingham
18	Hampstead	Sunderland
19	Liverpool	Wandsworth
20	Rochdale	Central Birmingham

The bottom five districts are:

	UPA	Townsend
1	East Yorkshire	East Surrey
2	East Surrey	South West Surrey
3	Wycombe	Wycombe
4	East Hertfordshire	West Surrey and North East Hampshire
5	Mid-Surrey	Mid-Surrey

about as high as the highest in England and Wales, but they have not been ranked with those in England and Wales as the Scottish data are published on the basis of post code sectors which have roughly the same populations as electoral wards in England and Wales but have a greater variation of populations. Ward maps have been drawn of UPA scores for a number of areas in England and Wales, and also for the post code sectors of Scotland (excluding the ethnic variable). One of these is illustrated in Figure 6.2 for the wards of Cleveland. The distribution of values of the UPA scores for the wards in England and Wales is shown in Figure 6.3.

Table 6.5 *Wards with the highest UPA scores*

	Ward name	District	UPA score
1	Brookhouse	Blackburn	72.95
2	Cathedral	Blackburn	72.89
3	University	Bradford	72.33
4	Spitalfields	Tower Hamlets	68.64
5	Wycliffe	Leicester	67.09
6	Carlton	Brent	67.03
7	Birmingham (Ladywood)	Birmingham	65.69
8	Birmingham (Aston)	Birmingham	64.37
9	Soho and Victoria	Sandwell	63.63
10	Birmingham (Deritend)	Birmingham	62.96
11	Birmingham (Duddeston)	Birmingham	62.57
12	Abercromby	Liverpool	62.25
13	Little Horton	Bradford	61.43
14	Birmingham (Sparkbrook)	Birmingham	61.12
15	Birmingham (Soho)	Birmingham	61.06
16	St Mary's	Tower Hamlets	61.01
17	Moss Side	Manchester	60.83
18	Foleshill	Coventry	60.78
19	Hulme	Manchester	58.76
20	Derby	Bolton	58.42

The UPA score method of assessing general practitioners' opinions was also used with a national sample of health visitors (and the district nurses in one District Health Authority). The nurses' survey gave very similar results to those obtained from general practitioners. The method is useful for primary care workers because

(1) it is geared towards the opinions of primary care workers nationally
(2) it is applicable to all areas, not just conventionally accepted inner cities
(3) it is more appropriate than consultation rates or any currently available measures of morbidity.

One of the drawbacks of the method is that it is based on the 1981 census data and can only be updated when the census is repeated in 1991. However, a comparison of scores for the boroughs of London based on 1971 and 1981 data shows that the general pattern of borough scores was maintained between these censuses.

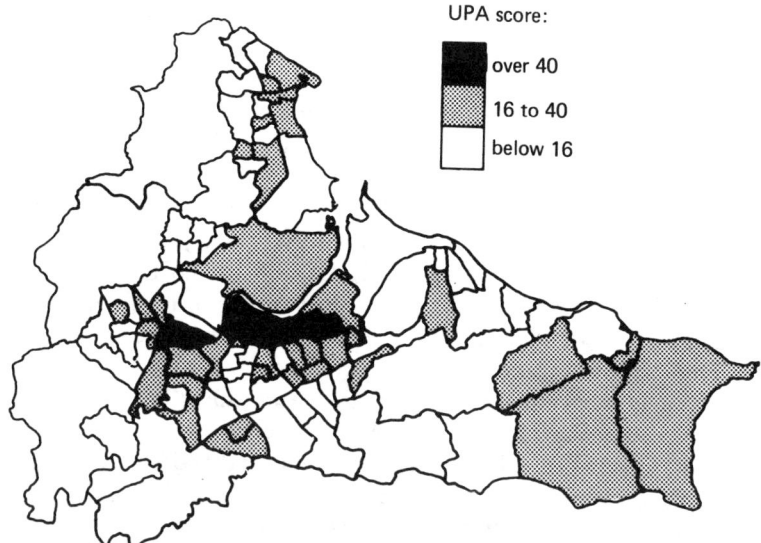

Figure 6.2 UPA score for the Cleveland wards.

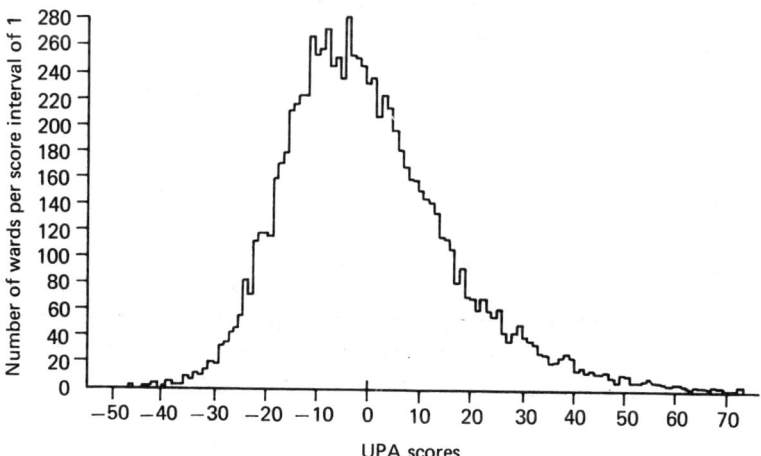

Figure 6.3 The distribution of values of the UPA scores for the wards in England and Wales (From: Jarman B. (1984). Underprivileged areas: validation and distribution of scores. *Br. Med. J.*, **289**, 1589, with permission.)

SOCIAL FACTORS, HEALTH AND HEALTH SERVICES

It can be shown that two of the variables which contribute to the UPA score (the proportions of *unemployed* and *unskilled*) correlate very strongly with SMRs and even more strongly with SMRs to age 75 or 65 years. In a multiple regression analysis it can be shown that these two variables explain 72% of the variation of SMRs to age 65 years for the District Health Authorities of England. They also correlate strongly with morbidity variables such as the proportions of temporarily and permanently sick and the proportion of low birth weight babies. These variables are measures of material deprivation and it is clear that they are strongly associated with the available measures of the levels of *illness* in different areas. Golborne Ward, for example, has a UPA score of 52.87 (putting it 54th from the top in England and Wales) and has higher than average levels of unemployment and unskilled workers (as well as other variables). Its SMR to age 65 years was 150 in 1985, 50% above the value which would be expected if national mortality rates were applied to the ward.

Other variables in the UPA score which are connected with *home conditions* and the availability of people to look after sick members of the family at home (the proportions of elderly living alone and of single parent and overcrowded households and unskilled workers) correlate more strongly with the usage of hospital inpatient and outpatient services. Using the last three of these variables it is possible to explain about 52% of the variation of hospital admission rates (standardized for age and sex). As hospital services account for 68% of NHS costs (as opposed to 7% for general practitioners), these social factors also correlate with areas where NHS district health authorities are under financial stress. This is because currently there is no allowance for the influence of social factors related to home conditions in hospital resource allocation nationally (although there is an allowance for illness levels as account is taken of full age range SMRs).

It is seen that components of the UPA score provide proxies for both illness levels and home conditions in different areas of the country. Where both of these dimensions of the UPA score are high, primary care workers are likely to be under stress and the health authorities in which they work are likely to have above average financial problems if adequate allowance is not made for home conditions in hospital resource allocation.

CHARACTERISTICS OF INNER CITY PRIMARY CARE SERVICES

Social factors not only affect health (through an association with morbidity and mortality, smoking rates, poor diet, failure to take up preventive services such as immunizations, and poor environmental conditions such as sanitation) but also have a major influence on the way health *care* is provided (see Chapter 3).

Looking at the *community medicine* aspect of health services in Inner London – especially health visitors and home nurses – the actual number of nurses per head of the population is roughly the same as that in Outer London and in England and Wales, although there are quite wide variations from area to area. The major difference is the percentage of these nurses attached to general practices, which is the lowest in the country for Inner London. These nurses tend to be younger, have less training and spend less time in post than those away from the city centre. There is some doubt expressed by nursing managers regarding the appropriateness of attachments to general practitioners in inner city areas, partly because of the lack of group practices and partly because of the lack of adequate general practitioner premises for the nurses to work from. There are also difficulties attracting nurses to work in areas where their expenses are high and patients have predominantly social and psychiatric problems for which their normal hospital training may not have prepared them.

One of the factors characterizing *general practice* in many inner city areas, and in Inner London particularly, is a predominance of elderly, single-handed general practitioners often practising from inadequate premises. As the incidence of the adverse social conditions increases, so these characteristics of general practice become more predominant (see Figure 6.4). Difficulties with traffic and parking make home visits more time consuming. The expenses of living and working in inner city areas are generally higher and there is no allowance for this in general practitioners' terms of service either in the form of an allowance similar to the London Allowance, which all other health service workers receive, or in the allowances for the employment of staff (rural areas have special rural practice payments to allow for difficulties in visiting). Similarly, the limits for the cost rent scheme to provide general practitioner premises are national ones with no regional differences to take account of the regional variation of costs of premises.

The Medical Practices Committee, which controls the distribution of

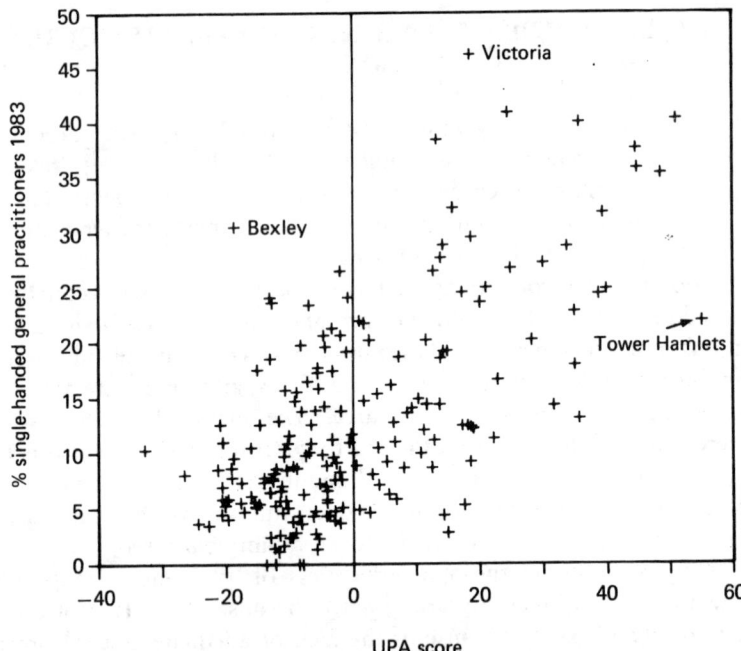

Figure 6.4 UPA scores versus per cent single-handed general practitioners in District Health Authorities, England, 1983.

general practitioners throughout the country, judges the need for additional general practitioners only by the average size of general practitioners' lists in the area under consideration. General practitioners' list sizes are slightly lower in inner city areas and hence there is no allowance by the Medical Practices Committee for the difficulties of practising in inner cities. Even worse, if general practitioners are keeping lower than average list sizes (perhaps to enable them to deal with above average workloads), then no new doctors are allowed to enter the area. Consequently, the average age of general practitioners in these areas increases and young trainees are unable to get in to practise. There is then the paradoxical situation of patients starving in the midst of plenty – patients can have difficulties getting onto general practitioners' lists despite there being apparently enough general practitioners according to the Medical Practices Committee rules based on list sizes (see p. 12).

THE 1987 GOVERNMENT WHITE PAPER

The proposals in the White Paper on improving primary health care services could prove to be very helpful for inner city general practice. The resources to be devoted to primary health care are to rise in real terms, additional revenue will be raised and a strategic shift in emphasis towards primary health care is to be implemented. This will be aimed at making services more responsive to consumers' needs and at giving them more choice, raising standards of care, promoting health and preventing illness. Although there are reservations about a number of proposals (such as the introduction of charges for eye testing), and many of the necessary details are as yet missing, overall there is a good chance that these objectives will be met. The consultation process following the Green Paper which was published in April 1986 showed that people are particularly interested in accessible, effective and sympathetic primary health care services, in prevention and health promotion, more information, the needs of the elderly and in the problems of deprived inner city and isolated rural areas. Many of these problems have been tackled in the recommendations that have been made and of these the following could be very helpful for inner cities in particular.

(1) The introduction of an inner city *Deprived Areas Allowance.* To implement this it will be necessary to have an accepted way of identifying the areas to which the allowance will apply, and the UPA score could be used for this. The allowance is very important because it will enable general practitioners working in deprived areas to receive a similar gross income to their colleagues working in other areas for a similar workload. To be entirely equitable, the reimbursement of expenses should also be related to the costs of living (as general practitioners must live near their patients) and working in an area.

(2) A *registration fee for preventive work* for patients aged over five years. This will be helpful because inner city areas have a higher turnover of patients and correspondingly more administrative work. The preventive medicine aspect will be particularly useful in working class areas where there is a lower uptake of cervical smears etc. and higher levels of smoking.

(3) Differential and *increased cost rent allowances* for inner cities and arrangements to make funds available for these developments in deprived areas if private sector funds are not available.

(4) *Modification of the Medical Practices Committee rules* based on local information, especially in inner cities.

(5) A *retirement age of 70 years* for general practitioners. Table 6.1 shows that there are more elderly general practitioners in Inner London, and the same applies to many other inner urban areas. There is no shortage of young trainees looking for posts in general practice and they are more likely than their older colleagues to have been trained specifically for general practice and for working in primary care teams.

(6) Possible *removal of the restriction that a general practitioner can employ only two members of ancillary staff.* However, the recommendation implies that there will be control of the number of ancillary staff at a Family Practitioner Committee level, and there may be cash limits on the numbers of ancillary staff that can be employed within a Family Practitioner Committee area.

(7) Making *Family Practitioner Committees responsible for establishing group practices* in deprived areas and also for making improvements in *premises* in these areas. Implemented properly, this recommendation in conjunction with a number of others could be of major importance. The establishment of primary care teams in good premises was probably the major recommendation of the Acheson Report.

(8) The introduction of a system more related to *medical and social needs* and the creation of *new vacancies where workloads are high* in relation to list sizes. This is a recommendation which could be difficult to administer because of the problems, discussed above, involved in measuring workloads and defining and measuring medical and social needs. It has been indicated, however, that these are not insuperable and there are methods which, although not perfect, are probably better than doing nothing.

The problems of inner city primary care are complex but it seems that there is to be a serious attempt to tackle them in an imaginative and comprehensive way.

FURTHER READING

Jarman B. (1981). *A Survey of Primary Care in London.* Occasional Paper 16. London: Royal College of General Practitioners.

Jarman B. (1983). Identification of underprivileged areas. *Br. Med. J.*, **286**, 1705.

Jarman B. (1984). Underprivileged areas: validation and distribution of scores. *Br. Med. J.*, **289**, 1589.

London Health Planning Consortium, Primary Health Care Study Group (Acheson Report; 1981). *Primary Health Care in Inner London.* London: DHSS.

Secretaries of State for Social Services, Wales, Northern Ireland and Scotland (White Paper on Primary Health Care, Cm. 249; 1987). *Promoting Better Health. The Government's Programme for Improving Primary Health Care.* London: HMSO.

Chapter

7

The Consultation

CONSULTATION SKILLS • CONSULTATION DATA • THE
DIAGNOSTIC PROCESS • THE DOCTOR-PATIENT
RELATIONSHIP

*The Art of Caring for the Patient
is Caring for the Patient*

CONSULTATION SKILLS

One of the major difficulties for students and trainees entering general
practice is to accommodate the different pathology with which they are
presented. Patients seen in hospitals have been highly selected and
present their symptoms in a reasonably well organized manner. In the
context of general practice, however, many patients present with
apparently unconnected and undifferentiated problems. If the doctor
attempts to formulate a diagnosis as he has been traditionally taught he
may well find himself frustrated, and the patient may begin to feel that
he is not being understood. The *consultation in* general practice is both
qualitatively and quantitatively different from the *history taking* model
that most medical students have been taught. The consultation
involves:

(1) *Interviewing skills*: the ability to establish a relationship with the
    patient enabling him to tell his story in his own words.
(2) *History taking skills*: questioning skills for obtaining specific
    information necessary for the doctor to make an appropriate
    decision concerning the management of the patient's problems. It
    is not always necessary – nor is it always possible – to arrive at a
    diagnosis in the classical way that is essential in hospital work.

(3) *Physical examination skills*: carrying out the necessary physical examination which may range from no examination at all to a full physical. It is not unusual for the doctor to use the physical examination to facilitate the first two elements of the consultation.

(4) *Problem-solving skills*: not all consultations will end in a prescription or referral. This is probably the second most difficult lesson to learn for the new entrant in general practice. The doctor will need to learn when to advise, when to reassure, when to investigate, when to 'treat' and when to do nothing.

In hospital medicine one is often told: 'don't just stand there, do something' – whereas in general practice more often than not one should remember: 'don't just do something, *stand there*'.

'Standing there' with the patient can be difficult and frustrating, and may not be what the young doctor thought his job was about. General practice will require the doctor to be able to tolerate a certain amount of uncertainty, and it is this ability which will allow him to maintain his enthusiasm for his work.

CONSULTATION DATA

Definitions

What do people do about their symptoms?

Fortunately for the NHS and the general practitioner, the majority of the population cope with their symptoms on their own. Figure 7.1 and Table 7.1 give some indication of how selective are the group of patients who ultimately consult their doctor. Patients who are seen in hospital form only a very small section, but because the accident and emergency department is often the meeting point between general practice and hospital medicine, students will often form their first impression of general practice from the group of patients who have failed to get satisfaction from their general practitioner. Thus, although this group is fairly small, it can influence for ever the student's notions of the quality of care in general practice.

How often do people see their general practitioner?

On average, two thirds of the population see their general practitioner at least once a year. However, as Figure 7.2 shows, a substantial

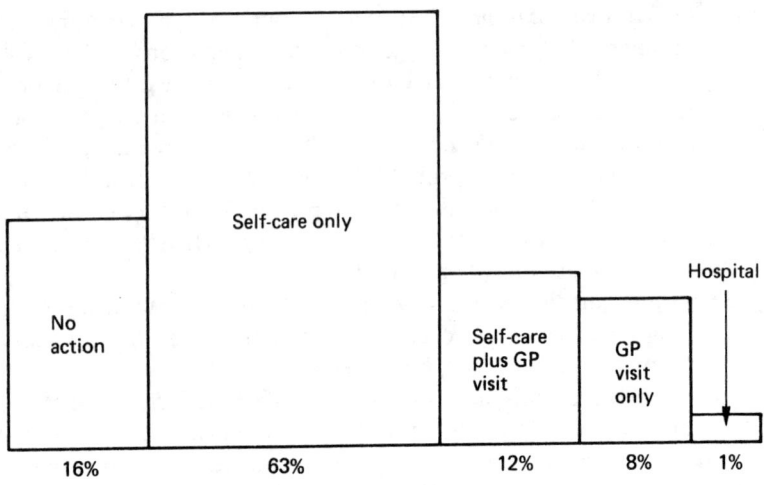

Figure 7.1 What people do about their symptoms.

Table 7.1 *Proportion of the population with symptoms and the proportion of general practice consultations by disease category*

Disease category	Symptoms[1] (%)	Consultations[2] (%)
Respiratory	26	33
Mental	21	15
Rheumatic	15	10
Digestive	11	11
Central nervous system	8	5
Skin	5	12
Cardiovascular	4	10
Other	10	4

Sources: [1]Wadsworth et al. (1971). [2]Fry (1973).

minority (the young, aged, socially disadvantaged) will seek help from their general practitioner fairly frequently throughout the year.

The majority of consultations now take place in the general practice

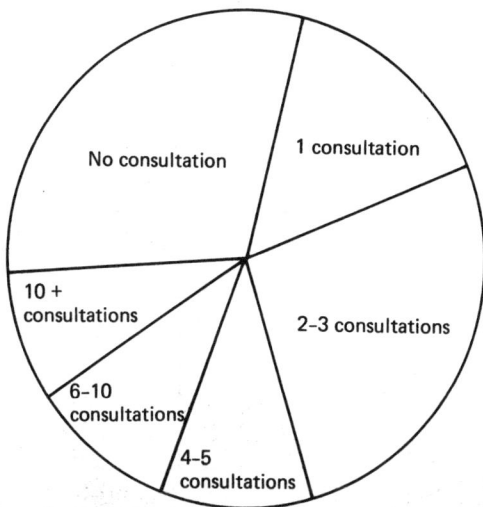

Figure 7.2 Yearly general practitioner consultations (UK, 1977). Proportions of adult patients (aged 16+) consulting various numbers of times. The average is 3–3.5 consultations per patient per year. (From Ritchie J. et al. 1981.)

premises and the rate of home visiting has fallen from 20–23% (1965) to about 12% (1981).

It is clear from Figure 7.3 that more women consult their doctors than men, and that the elderly, the young and socio-economic groups IV and V consult more frequently. The latter fact is of some importance to the young doctor, who if not by birth then by education will belong to the socio-economic group that consults the doctor least. The beliefs, values and language that the doctor brings to his work may well diminish his ability to help the patient whose own background and culture may be very different.

Consultation and time

Probably no other factor causes as much concern and comment as the *length* of the consultation. Studies suggest that general practitioners spend over half their working time consulting. On average, a general practitioner will see between 120–150 patients a week, and the average

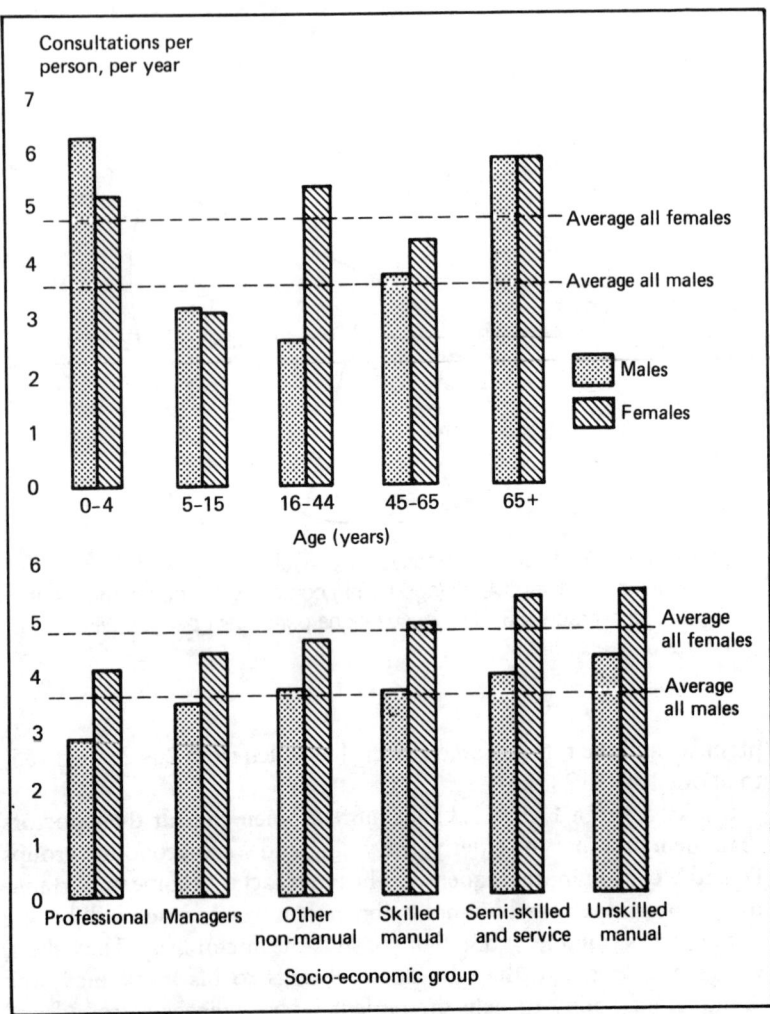

Figure 7.3 Patient consultations by selected groups, Great Britain 1980. (From Office of Population Censuses and Surveys 1984.)

consultation time is about eight minutes although there are moves to increase this to ten minutes as list sizes are reducing. It has been argued that this short time is woefully inadequate for a proper assessment of the patient's problems. The realities are that general practitioners are able to determine their own time framework and can prolong consultation times to well beyond 15 minutes if required. Similarly it is possible to see patients relatively frequently during the course of a week and it is a common observation that two 10-minute consultations spaced by a day or two are often more productive than one 20-minute consultation. Nevertheless it is clear that consultation times in general practice are unlikely to change greatly and the skills necessary to work within that framework are essential and basic to all general practitioners.

The literature of consultation analysis

Several authors have studied the consultation in general practice and formulated '*models*' that will allow the student to observe the process in a systematic manner. Some of these models are summarized below. **Byrne and Long** analysed 5000 audiotaped consultations and identified six *phases* which, although presented in a logical sequence, rarely occur in a systematic manner. These phases are:
(1) relating to the patient
(2) discovering the reason for the patient's attendance
(3) conducting a verbal or physical examination or both
(4) considering the patient's problems
(5) detailing treatment or further investigation
(6) terminating.
  Byrne and Long also identified seven different *styles* of consultation which ranged along a grid as shown below:

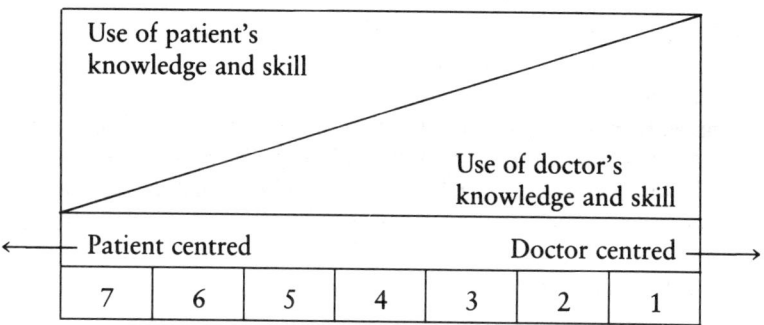

In a 'doctor-centred' consultation, the doctor was more likely to make a decision for the patient and instruct him to seek some service. In a 'patient-centred' consultation, the doctor was more likely to seek the patient's views and permit him to make his own decision concerning the outcome.

Stott and Davis, and also Gray (see below), outlined the *tasks* of the consultation and the process by which these tasks were carried out.

(a) Management of presenting problem	(b) Modification of help-seeking behaviour
(c) Management of continuing problem	(d) Opportunistic health promotion

Gray

Problem presented	Solution presented
Problem discussed and defined	Solution discussed and defined
Problem agreed with doctor	Solution agreed with patient

Pietroni explored the importance of *non-verbal communication* in the consultation. He observed that within any two-person interaction, over 70% of the communication occurring is channelled through the non-verbal band. Non-verbal behaviour allows the observer to discern the *emotional state* (i.e. a feeling or affect, such as happiness, anger, surprise, fear, disgust or sadness) that the communicator is experiencing at the moment. These feelings are usually communicated through facial expressions which are recognized and decoded by the observer. The degree of affect (*how* angry or sad) is more commonly communicated through posture. For example, a sad facial expression, limp shoulders, and drooping head would tend to indicate greater sadness than a sad face alone.

As well as communicating aspects of one's emotional state, non-verbal behaviour is indicative of *interpersonal attitudes*. The distance two people choose to put between themselves when conversing indicates something about their degree of intimacy and their relative status. How a doctor chooses to sit in relation to a patient, for example, indicates not only his perception of his status, but how he feels about the patient and how he feels about relating to the patient.

Non-verbal behaviour also gives certain *specific information* about the individual observed. Characteristics such as age, race, sex and social status can be reasonably determined through observation of physical appearance – hair style, clothes, bearing and posture.

Research studies in this area have now been undertaken in sufficient detail to allow us to begin thinking about practical applications. As far as the clinician is concerned, those areas of non-verbal behaviour which appear to be of greatest importance in establishing *rapport* are:

(1) *Eye contact* – an appropriate amount of direct eye contact with the patient is not only necessary to collect information, but appears to be an essential component of developing rapport.

(2) *Hand movement* – the amount of hand movement (either with pen or notes), as well as the nature of gesturing, influences the patient's perception of whether the doctor is listening or not.

(Both of these behaviours are affected by whether the physician is writing notes at the time of the interview. It is believed that writing and reading notes are distracting and create a distance between doctor and patient.)

(3) *Paralanguage* – the speech rate, fluency, and voice quality of a doctor's verbal communication is an important factor in determining the impact of the content. It is not what one says, it is how one says it. This well known phrase appears to be equally important in the interview between doctor and patient.

(4) *Proximity* – the space the doctor keeps between himself and the patient, as well as whether he is sitting or standing, influence the quality of the interaction. The habit of interviewing patients who are already undressed and on an examining table should be reduced to the absolute minimum. It is the blending of the ability to send and receive verbal and non-verbal cues that produces a sensitive clinician who, above all else, must be an effective communicator.

Not only should the physician concern himself with establishing rapport, he should also be able to observe and understand subtle cues the patient may be sending. The *cues* that appear to be of the most importance for the clinician are:

(1) *Facial expression* Does the patient have a characteristic facial expression (anger, sadness)?

(2) *Eye contact and gaze behaviour* What amount of eye contact does the patient use? Does his angle of gaze change? Are there frequent gaze shifts?

(3) *Posture and position* Where does the patient choose to sit? What posture does he adopt? Does this change and if so when?

(4) *Gestures* Does the patient use head nods and if so, when? Are his hands still or moving? Does he gesture with his hand around his mouth?

(5) *Clothes* Is the patient's clothing appropriate? Does it indicate anything about his personality?

(6) *Speech rate, tone, and inflection* Is the speech rate rapid, or slow? Is the pitch flat? Are any words slurred? Is there an inflection on parts of the content?

(7) *Non-fluencies* How many hesitations, pauses, slips of the tongue etc. are there? Is there a mumbling or sentence change around a particular topic?

(8) *Non-verbal vocalizations* Does the patient cough, sneeze, clear his throat, gasp or sigh audibly? If so, when?

The observation of non-verbal behaviour during the interview gives the doctor an opportunity to make assessments and provisional hypotheses with much more certainty and at an earlier stage of the diagnostic process. It facilitates the interaction between doctor and patient, and it shortens the diagnostic process. It helps to avoid unnecessary investigations, and it enhances the therapeutic process.

Pendleton explored the importance of health beliefs and described the cycle of care involved in consultations. The '*antecedents*' to a consultation are factors that help to shape it. These antecedents include the expectations, values and health beliefs of both doctor and patient. Pendleton identified a set of *tasks* which he felt the doctor needs to achieve. Like Byrne's 'phases' of a consultation, these tasks – although set out in a logical sequence – are rarely tackled in this order:

Tasks of the consultation

(1) To define the reason for the patient attending
(2) To consider other problems (continuing problems, at risk factors)
(3) To choose with the patient an appropriate action for each problem
(4) To achieve a shared understanding of the problems with the patient
(5) To involve the patient in the management and encourage him to accept appropriate responsibility
(6) To use time and resources appropriately

(7) To establish and maintain a relationship which helps to achieve the other tasks.

Balint did not use systematic behavioural concepts to analyse consultations but his work has been of great influence to general practitioners. His psycho-analytic background enabled him to explain the mechanics of a consultation in a manner that has not been bettered since his seminal work *The Doctor, the Patient and the Illness* (1958). Balint was the first to bring doctors' attention to the importance of the doctor-patient relationship, and several of his observations now form the basis for the training of vocational trainees. These observations include:

(1) *The doctor as a 'drug'* The doctor is the most often 'prescribed' intervention in consultations, i.e. his ability to advise, reassure and listen could be seen as 'drugs' that are prescribed, and the doctor needs to learn the right 'dose' and side-effects of these prescriptions.

(2) *The doctor's own feelings* Probably Balint's greatest contribution was to draw attention to the importance of the doctor's own feelings during a consultation. These feelings, which traditionally most doctors have been taught to deny or avoid, can be – in Balint's view – very helpful both for the patient and the doctor. Balint identified how the emotional state of the patient (anger, depression, fear) can often be transferred to the doctor – and of course vice versa. Balint training involved the capacity to use these feelings both as diagnostic and therapeutic tools.

(3) *The underlying reason* Balint observed that, more often than not, the patient's presenting complaint is not the real reason for attending and may be viewed as a 'ticket to get through the door'. The doctor will need to develop the skills required to uncover the 'real' reason if he is to help the patient.

Discovering the underlying reason may require a willingness to enquire into the psychological and emotional areas of a patient's life. The skills that are required for this aspect of the consultation are different from those needed when asking about a physical symptom. It must be said that many doctors who take to the Balint model of consulting run into the danger of confusing emotional curiosity with caring, and it is not always necessary or helpful to adopt a style that can be experienced as an invasion by the patient.

Establishing goals

Each consultation may have a different *purpose* which will affect the way it develops. The first consultation with a new patient will be different from one where the doctor knows the patient well. The doctor's 'goal' may differ from the patient's, and communication difficulties will arise if the differences are not recognized sooner rather than later.

Harris has outlined ten main reasons for patients consulting:
(1) For relief of symptoms, and/or for diagnosis
(2) For some other normal medical service
(3) For official recognition of sickness, e.g. certification
(4) For follow-up requested by the doctor himself
(5) For access to other parts of the health and welfare services
(6) For drugs on which the patient is dependent
(7) As habitual response to anxieties
(8) For support and recognition
(9) For playing games and acting out dramas
(10) For more than one of the above.

Keeping in mind these reasons why the patient is consulting is important throughout; nevertheless, it is helpful to have three general goals in mind before commencing any consultation.

Goal 1 – Creating and establishing a relationship

Rapport, or the quality of human contact, in a consultation is like the lubricant in complex machinery. Without it, the machine ceases to function; with it, the machine proceeds uninterrupted.

Establishing rapport is more than just being friendly. It requires a demonstration of active, concerned interest in the patient. It necessitates the creation of an atmosphere which enables the patient to feel secure and accepted. James Spence describes the *unit of medical practice* as 'the occasion when, in the intimacy of the consulting room, a person who is ill or believes himself to be ill seeks the advice of a doctor whom he trusts.' The words *intimacy* and *trust* invoke the notion of the consulting room as a 'safe space'. The atmosphere created by the architecture, the furniture, lighting, the position of the desk, those personal possessions displayed, all help to create a sense of ease – or, conversely, a sense of 'dis-ease'. It is worth spending a few moments before meeting the patient and ensuring familiarity with the patient's name. Being aware of whether the patient is expecting to see someone else can be very important in establishing a relationship and helps to anticipate the patient's initial response.

Greeting Each of us will develop our own form of greeting which feels natural and comfortable. Some of the important factors in the initial stages of the consultation, especially with a new patient, include mentioning both the *patient's* and *your own name*, and *who you are* (e.g. 'I am a fourth-year medical student and have been asked to see you. . . .'). *Good eye contact*, and if you can manage a *smile*, will help to enhance the human qualities which are so necessary to aid medical exchange. Shaking hands as a form of greeting has largely gone out of fashion, but with new patients or elderly patients it may well serve to 'break the ice'.

Making the patient comfortable The majority of consultations in general practice will take place in the doctor's consulting room. Seeing patients in their own homes or in hospital (wards, outpatients) will alter the setting and require the doctor to adjust his style. Where the patient sits and how the chairs are placed in relation to the desk influences the quality of the communication possible between doctor and patient.

Taking notes Most students taking a history try to write down everything the patient has said. Part of the task of any consultation is to keep a record of it but taking notes not only breaks eye contact, which may be important, but also prevents the doctor from observing the patient's face and hands for subtle, non-verbal clues. It is helpful to get into the habit of jotting down any important dates or details, but leave the writing up of notes until after the patient has left.

Goal 2 – Obtaining information relating to the patient's problems

In obtaining information from the patient, it is necessary to be aware of certain skills and techniques that are helpful in carrying out this task. In the same way as turning a patient on his left side is helpful when listening for mitral diastolic murmur, it is also helpful to use certain 'techniques' to elicit information during the consultation. These are the skills of the interview and, like all skills, will only improve with practice.

These skills can be divided into three categories, although the division between them is by no means clear cut.

(1) *Avoiding habits which block communication*
   (a) *General attitude*
     – patronizing role affectation
     – tenseness, nervousness
     – coldness, unfriendliness
     – defensiveness
     – appearance of being uninterested, too relaxed or casual
   (b) *Specific behaviours*
     – use of jargon
     – failure to use the patient's language
     – inability to keep quiet
     – taking notes too elaborately
     – interrupting the patient
     – lack of a purposeful direction in the interview
     – making unwarranted assumptions
     – giving advice too early
     – allowing personal emotions to get in the way
(2) *Use of basic skills to obtain information the patient is willing to give*
   (a) *Questioning*
     – open-ended questions
     – facilitating techniques – verbal and non-verbal
     – simple probing
     – reflected questions
   (b) *Active listening*
     – restatement
     – clarification
     – empathy
     – summarizing
   (c) *Non-verbal awareness*
     – cues relating to interaction with the interviewer
     – cues relating to the emotional state of the interviewee
     – cues relating to a 'personal statement' of the interviewee
(3) *Use of more advanced skills to push for resistant information*
   – confrontation
   – use of silence
   – interpretations
   – deeper probing
   – interpretation of more subtle, non-verbal communication of the patient
   – use of touch

Goal 3 – Conveying appropriate information to the patient about his problem

It is important to allow sufficient time for this task to be adequately completed in the interview. All too often, the patient is left not knowing what decision has been made concerning the probable diagnosis, further investigations, referral or treatment.

A useful habit to adopt is trying to clarify early on in the consultation what the ending is likely to involve (i.e. certificate, prescription, referral). One of the important early lessons in general practice is to realize that not everything needs to be completed within one consultation. Apart from the few urgent and acute medical problems, asking the patient to come back can avoid your 'rushing' the ending and can allow both you and the patient some thinking space. It will also ensure that you do not keep your next patient waiting too long.

It is helpful to indicate to the patient, usually non-verbally, that the consultation is about to end and to give him an opportunity to ask any final questions. In a proportion of consultations, this may lead to a 'By the way doctor, while I am here. . . .' and you may find yourself starting on a new round of questions having already spent 15 minutes. The 'By the way . . .' may include the most important reason for attending and you may have no choice but to start again. More often than not, however, it is possible to suggest that the patient returns for a further consultation.

THE DIAGNOSTIC PROCESS

It is relatively easy to dissect the consultation into a series of behavioural *techniques* and interviewing gambits and to forget what medicine is all about (just as it is possible to focus on the pathophysiology of the presenting problem and forget about the person). Throughout any consultation, the student/doctor has to juggle with different sets of information, some coming directly from the patient, some the result of the doctor's observations and some from investigative procedures. The doctor has to arrive at a conclusion and, if he is versed in the hospital-model of history taking, he may feel obliged to arrive at a diagnosis before he can proceed with treatment. Yet treatment starts the moment the patient seeks the help of a doctor. The effectiveness of the treatment offered, whether it be pills, advice or surgery, may be determined by factors present even before the patient enters the consulting room – his own expectations and health beliefs (e.g. 'my cold will not get better unless I have an antibiotic', or 'I had to wait 25 minutes to see the doctor and he lost my notes, so I won't comply with his instructions').

The notion that a diagnosis must be arrived at 'objectively' and that it must occur before treatment are hallmarks of what has been labelled the *bio-medical model*. The diagnostic process in general practice cannot be seen as a separate activity and it is clear from observing consultations how much treatment is achievable even when no diagnosis is made. A general practitioner faced with a young girl with right-sided abdominal pain on a home visit has to make the decision to leave her at home or to admit her to hospital. Whether she has appendicitis or not may be only part of this decision; all sorts of other factors will be taken into account – the level of anxiety, home circumstances, who is on call, the doctor's own level of confidence etc. The surgeon examining this young girl in the accident and emergency department will need to make a more precise decision – 'do I operate or not' – and the amount of information he requires to make this decision is in a more specialized and narrow domain. Similarly, the pathologist who examines the removed appendix has to decide whether there is any inflammation in the specimen. All three doctors have to decide whether the diagnosis of appendicitis is correct, but each arrives at this decision using different levels of information. The first doctor, by allowing both objective and subjective as well as psychosocial data to enter into his decision making process, has strayed from the classical 'scientific' bio-medical model into what has been labelled the *bio-psychosocial model*. It is increasingly clear that, for most general practitioners, the bio-psychosocial model provides for a more complete framework in which to undertake a consultation. It allows the doctor to deal with the notion of 'feeling unwell' with no organic disease. It allows clarification between the notions of 'health' and 'sickness', as these are so clearly influenced by psychological, cultural and social factors.

Arriving at a diagnosis using the bio-medical model entails obtaining as much information as possible (history taking, physical examination, investigation) and not entertaining a diagnosis until all the data are collected, e.g. a patient presenting with a headache may require extensive investigation, including a brain scan, before the doctor feels able to exclude a diagnosis of brain tumour.

Using the bio-psychosocial model, not only is the quality and quantity of information collected different but so is the diagnostic process. Rather than follow a linear pathway of deductive reasoning, the doctor will use his sense of 'pattern recognition' and come up with a probable hypothesis for the cause of the headache which he will then proceed to test, e.g. most headaches are caused by tension/anxiety – let me check whether that may be the cause by asking a 'discriminate question'; if the answer is negative, then let me entertain a different hypothesis – and so on. *Pattern recognition, hypothesis testing* and *discriminate questions* appear to be the hallmarks of expert clinicians whether they use the bio-medical or the bio-psychosocial model.

THE DOCTOR-PATIENT RELATIONSHIP

Central to the consultation is the quality of the relationship that develops between doctor and patient. We have already emphasized the importance of rapport or empathy and, to reiterate the opening quotation, 'the art of caring for the patient is caring for the patient.' Yet it can at times be particularly difficult to care for the patient. We may not ourselves be in a caring mood or the patient may not be someone we find particularly sympathetic – he may even remind us of a figure in our personal life with whom we may have difficulty.

The relationship between doctor and patient can develop along several different lines; Szasz and Hollender identified the three most common:

(1) *Active-passive* – the patient is the passive recipient of the doctor's expertise and wisdom. The doctor possesses all the skill and the patient needs only 'allow' the doctor to proceed – e.g. treating a patient with a fracture, stroke or diabetic coma.

(2) *Guidance-cooperation* – here, the doctor acts more in the role of teacher or educator. He knows more about the condition and advises the patient as to what he or she should do. He requires the patient's cooperation, but all the patient needs to do is 'follow the doctor's orders', e.g. taking a course of antibiotics, following a diet or giving up smoking.

(3) *Mutual participation* – both doctor and patient are involved in the decision-making process, and the patient is allowed to arrive at the final decision on his or her own, e.g. whether to proceed with termination or sterilization.

On other occasions, it may be that the patient is the active partner in the relationship asking, or at times instructing, the doctor for what he or she wants. It is in such consultations that doctors may feel frustrated or angry. Being asked to prescribe antibiotics, refer to a specialist or give a certificate against one's better judgement, can create much tension within any consultation. It is at times such as these that the doctor has to ask himself whether his need to remain 'in charge' is always in the patient's best interest.

Central to whatever relationship develops between doctor and patient — and all those described may well be appropriate at any one time — is the question of *trust*. The consultation is a complex activity requiring not only the knowledge and skills described in this chapter but also an attitude which allows for the essential uniqueness of the human aspects of an interaction to emerge.

REFERENCES AND FURTHER READING

Balint M. (1958). *The Doctor, His Patient and the Illness.* London: Tavistock Publications.

Byrne P., Long B. (1976). *Doctors Talking to Patients.* London: HMSO.

Fry J. (1973). *Self-care: its Place in the Total Health Care System.* Report by an independent working party, September 1973 (mimeographed).

Gray D. P. (1982). *Training for General Practice.* Plymouth: Macdonald & Evans Publications.

Harris C. (1984). *The Doctor-Patient Relationship.* Edinburgh: Churchill Livingstone.

Pendleton D. (1984). *The Consultation.* Oxford: Oxford University Press.

Office of Population Censuses and Surveys (1984). *General Household Survey 1982.* London: HMSO.

Pietroni P. C. (1976). Language and communication. In *General Practice* (Tanner B., ed) pp. 162–79. London: Hodder & Stoughton.

Ritchie J., Jacoby A., Bone M. (1981). *Access to Primary Health Care.* London: HMSO.

Stott N. C. H., Davis R. H. (1979). The exceptional potential in each primary care consultation. *J. Royal Coll. Gen. Practit.,* **29**, 201.

Szasz T., Hollender M. (1956). Basic models of doctor-patient relationships. *Arch. Int. Med.,* **97**, 585.

Wadsworth M. E. J., Blamey R., Butterfield W. J. H. (1971). *Health and Sickness: the Choice of Treatment*. London: Tavistock Publications.

White A. (1953). The patient sits down. *Psychosomat. Med.*, 3, 4.

Williamson J. D., Donaher K. (1978). *Self-Care in Health*. Bromley: Croom Helm.

Chapter

8

Prescribing in General Practice

GENERAL DATA ON PRESCRIBING • THE SELECTED LIST • PRACTICAL DETAILS FOR PRESCRIBING

A significant part of the work of a general practitioner is associated with prescribing for his or her patients – a prescription is given in 78% of consultations. The apothecaries were the predecessors of general practitioners and, until 1829, they were allowed to charge only for the prescriptions which they gave, not for their consultations; hence, a tradition of giving prescriptions at consultations was built up and some of this may have persisted to the present day.

GENERAL DATA ON PRESCRIBING

About 84% of all drug costs in the NHS are for drugs prescribed by general practitioners and dispensed from the *Pharmaceutical Services* part of the Family Practitioner Services. In England in 1984–5, the prescriptions written by general practitioners cost £1500 million (11% of the total NHS costs), while the services of the general practitioners themselves (the *General Medical Services* part of the Family Practitioner Services) cost a little less than £1000 million (7%). About £1000 million was also spent on over-the-counter pharmaceutical products without NHS prescriptions (see Table 9.2, p. 157 for details of the commonest categories of drugs to which this applies). About 6% of general practitioner prescribed drugs are dispensed by *dispensing doctors* – general practitioners who are permitted to dispense for patients who live more than a mile from a chemist and hence have difficulty obtaining their drugs (these patients are on the general practitioner's 'dispensing list'). Pharmacists are paid from the *Prescription Pricing Authority* which deals with all NHS general practitioner prescriptions, and their own remuneration is about a quarter of the cost of the Pharmaceutical Services. General practitioners are given an annual analysis of their prescribing costs and those whose average prescription costs per patient, after allowing for differences in the age profile of their patients, are more than 25% above their local Family Practitioner Committee average costs are visited by DHSS regional medical officers to discuss these costs.

The list of drugs that can be prescribed is given in the *Drug Master Index* which contains over 20 000 preparations if all strengths of drugs are included as well as appliances (a drug is a substance which can alter the structure or function of a living organism). In a study carried out in the Department of General Practice at St Mary's Hospital Medical School of the prescribing habits of 50 local general practitioners over a period of two years, we found that the average general practitioner uses 300 to 500 drugs, and that the 50 general practitioners together used a little over 2000 drugs (including all formulations) during the two years.

The total number of prescriptions dispensed (meaning prescription items of which there are on average 1.63 per prescription form) has increased from 4.5 to 7.0 per person per year between 1949 and 1986. This rise is partly due to an increase in the proportion of those over pensionable age in the population (for whom the average was 15 items prescribed per person per year in 1985). On average in 1981–2, patients consulted their general practitioners between 3.4 and 4.3 times per year according to two different studies carried out at that time. Each patient received about 6.7 prescription items on 4.1 prescription forms. If a prescription is given at about 78% of all consultations, this implies that between 23% and 55% of all prescriptions which patients receive in general practice are given without the patient seeing the general practitioner at a consultation. These are called *repeat prescriptions* and are generally for long-term treatments, e.g. for epilepsy or myxoedema, but are sometimes given for other illnesses for which it would be desirable for the general practitioner to see the patient.

Computers are now used by some general practitioners to manage their repeat prescribing. These have the advantage of making sure that patients' treatments are well recorded and that prescriptions are written clearly, but they could encourage inappropriate use of repeat prescribing. Repeat prescriptions should not be given for tranquillizers or other drugs likely to lead to addiction. For physical illnesses, a date for review should be set for each prescription. In principle, computers that are used for prescribing could be programmed to convert the names of all drugs prescribed to their generic form. In May 1987, two companies which have developed computing systems for general practitioners (Abies and VAMP) announced that they would provide top-of-the-range computer systems for general practitioners effectively free of charge, including training, maintenance and updating, in exchange for computerized details of virtually all of their prescribing and the related diagnoses. This would enable drug companies to detect adverse reactions and help with post-marketing surveillance, and would also give them valuable market research data. The offer covers 3000 to 4000 practices and could make a significant impact on general practitioner prescribing and practice management.

The most common and most expensive *individual drugs* given by general practitioners in September 1985, in terms of frequency and cost of prescription, can be seen from Table 8.1. The commonest and most costly *therapeutic classes* of drugs in 1985 were, in rank order:

Most common drugs	*Most costly drugs*
Diuretics	Anti-inflammatory agents (non-steroid)
Heart preparations	Heart preparations
Topical skin preparations	Asthma preparations
Penicillins	Other gastrointestinal preparations (e.g. H_2 antagonists)
Asthma preparations	Antihypertensives
Anti-inflammatory agents (non-steroid)	Diuretics
Minor analgesics	Penicillins
Hypnotics	Topical skin preparations

These orders are constantly changing – for instance, the proportion of the total prescriptions in the sedatives and tranquillizers therapeutic group has decreased noticeably from first place in 1979 to ninth in 1985. Most of this reduction occurred after the introduction of the *selected list* (see below) of drugs in this group in 1985; there was a fall of one third in the number of prescriptions being written from 1982 to 1986. Nationally, the 20 most expensive individual drugs account for about 20% of the total drug bill. For an individual general practitioner, the 20 most expensive drugs which the general practitioner prescribes

Table 8.1 Drug economies using generic substitution or possible alternatives (England, September 1985)

Drug now given	Net ingredient cost (£1000s)	Alternative drug in some cases	Cost per tablet etc. Drug (p)	Cost per tablet etc. Alternative (p)	Ratio	Monthly possible saving (£1000)
Generic substitution						
Ventolin inhaler	1672	salbutamol inhaler	262.00	218.00	.832	281
Brufen 400 mg	809	ibuprofen 400 mg	6.07	3.10	.511	396
Zyloric 300 mg	676	allopurinol 100 mg × 3	38.93	14.25	.366	429
Aldomet 250 mg	474	methyldopa 250 mg	5.94	2.85	.480	247
Septrin	389	co-trimoxazole	10.55	5.60	.531	183
			Total maximum possibly monthly saving			1536
Possible alternative (in some cases only)						
Zantac 150 mg	1869	cimetidine 400 mg	45.72	29.66	.649	656
Moduretic	1173	Dyazide	8.80	6.32	.718	331
Tenormin 100 mg	1147	propranolol 160 mg	24.93	1.30	.052	1087
Feldene 10 mg	1009	indomethacin 25 mg × 1.5	15.00	1.50	.100	908
Naprosyn 500 mg	994	indomethacin	19.73	3.00	.152	843
Amoxil 250 mg	973	ampicillin 500 mg	16.60	6.73	.405	579
Tenoretic	931	propranolol 160+bendro 5	26.57	1.54	.058	877
atenolol 100 mg	812	propranolol 160 mg	24.93	1.30	.052	770
ranitidine 150 mg	763	cimetidine 400 mg	45.72	29.66	.649	268
Voltarol retard 100 mg	711	indomethacin 25 mg × 4	42.79	4.00	.093	645
Voltarol 50 mg	683	indomethacin 25 mg × 2	18.55	2.00	.108	609
Lederfen 300 mg	666	indomethacin 25 mg	17.98	1.00	.056	629
Indocid R 75 mg	663	indomethacin 25 mg × 3	28.57	3.00	.105	593
Inderal LA	500	propranolol 160 mg	23.79	1.30	.054	473
Minocin 50 mg	498	oxytetracycline 250 mg	24.24	1.70	.070	463
Naprosyn 250 mg	481	indomethacin 25 mg × 1.5	10.40	1.50	.144	412
Feldene 20 mg	457	indomethacin 25 mg × 3	30.00	3.00	.100	411
Slow Trasicor 160 mg	444	propranolol 160 mg	24.43	1.30	.053	420
Atenolol 50 mg	411	propranolol 80 mg	17.43	0.84	.048	391
Gaviscon liquid 500 ml	400	magnesium trisil 500 ml	288.00	50.00	.174	331
Tenormin LS 50 mg	376	propranolol 80 mg	17.43	0.84	.048	358
			Total maximum possible monthly saving			12 054

Total costs are about 28% above the net ingredient costs shown. Note that only in some circumstances, depending on the clinical situation, could the alternative drug be used.

Source: Department of Health and Social Security, Statistics and Research Division (1986). *Prescription Analysis for July 1986.* London: DHSS.

may account for about 40% of that general practitioner's prescription costs.

THE SELECTED LIST

In April 1985, a 'limited' or 'selected' list of drugs was introduced by the NHS for *seven* therapeutic groups – tranquillizers, hypnotics, minor analgesics, cough suppressants, antacids, laxatives and vitamins. This meant that only drugs from a selected list of mainly *generic* (as opposed to proprietary) preparations in these seven therapeutic groups could be used on NHS prescriptions. They were chosen on the basis of being medicines prescribed mainly for the relief of symptoms caused by *minor and self-limiting ailments* that do not normally call for medical intervention. The principle of a selected list of drugs could be extended to other classes of drugs, provided that it is based on the grounds of need, safety, efficiency (including convenience for the patient and doctor) and economy – i.e. to improve patient care and to economize in the use of drugs.

Extension of the selected list principle to cover other therapeutic classes would enable greater savings to be made, as shown in Table 8.1, for drugs such as indomethacin, ibuprofen, allopurinol, salbutamol, methyldopa, propranolol and so on. In view of the fact that the bioavailability of the active ingredients has to conform to set standards, it is possible – depending on the clinical situation – to substitute generic for proprietary drugs, or to use cheaper drugs when they would be equally satisfactory. Not only would this reduce the drugs budget but a selected list of drugs would mean that general practitioners would be using a smaller number of drugs, chosen on the grounds of need, safety, efficiency and economy, giving them a chance to get to know this selected list well. Some of the advantages and disadvantages of generic prescribing are summarized later in this chapter. A number of practices have introduced their own selected lists, and organizations such as the World Health Organization have drawn up basic lists of recommended drugs.

In the year ending February 1987, only 36% of general practice prescriptions were written using generic (non-proprietary) names. Drug companies are given 20 years *patent protection* for their drugs. Doctors may write prescriptions using the generic name and the pharmacist may dispense any brand of the drug, but the cost to the

NHS will be only the generic drug cost: this will be the same as the proprietary cost until the patent licence runs out when other cheaper versions will appear and the generic cost will be less. Drug companies employ thousands of representatives who visit doctors to tell them the benefits of the company's drugs, but the DHSS has only about ten regional medical officers (full-time equivalents) who are responsible for pointing out the need for economical prescribing. In answer to a Parliamentary Question, Kenneth Clarke stated that sales promotion expenses returned by large companies (sales over £2 million to the NHS) were £155.8 million in 1982 – about £5000 per general practitioner. From 1 April 1982, the limit on sales promotion expenditure was set at 9% of turnover under the *Pharmaceutical Price Regulation Scheme* – currently about £5000 per general practitioner. It would be easy to modify the prescription form to ensure that drugs were mostly dispensed in their generic form unless the general practitioner specifically indicated otherwise. This would still allow general practitioners the freedom to select a proprietary drug if they thought it necessary. The principle of generic substitution has been used in most NHS hospitals for some years.

A difficulty with the introduction of a selected list to cover all drugs which may be prescribed on the NHS, or adopting a system of mainly generic prescribing, is that either method would reduce the profits of drugs companies whose main income is not from generic drugs, and possibly lead to some unemployment. For these and other reasons this change could therefore be difficult to implement. On the other hand, it has been suggested that brand names stifle competition, and removing the protection which the industry now has would eventually lead to a healthier situation. The British pharmaceutical industry is generally considered to be successful, being responsible for the discovery of cimetidine and beta-blockers, for example. It is therefore necessary to strike a balance between keeping a healthy and successful industry – which is able to continue making significant therapeutic advances and keep its leading position in the world – and the apparent advantages of a selected list of drugs (or generic prescribing).

PRACTICAL DETAILS FOR PRESCRIBING

The following are some brief notes on practical aspects of prescribing in general practice.

(1) Reference works are:
   (a) The *British National Formulary* (BNF)
   (b) The *Drug & Therapeutics Bulletin* – an excellent publication from the Consumers' Association issued free to general practitioners (except in Scotland)
   (c) the *Merseyside Regional Drug Information Bulletin*
   (d) *Martindale*
   (e) *Prescribers' Journal* (often rather hospital orientated)
   (f) the *Monthly Index of Medical Specialties* (MIMS), which includes an index of generic (non-proprietary) drugs.

(2) Prescriptions are for *topical* (skin and mucous membranes), *enteral* (mouth and rectum), *parenteral* (injection) and *inhalation* drugs.

(3) The prescription should be written in ink/ball point and state:
   - the patient's name and address (and age if under 12)
   - the full drug name, dose and frequency of administration (in English)
   - the number of days' treatment to be dispensed (or total number or amount to be given for drugs that are to be taken as necessary). Use the box at the top of the NHS pad to give the number of days.

(4) For *controlled drugs*, the amount must be in words and figures and the prescription written in full in the doctor's handwriting (except for phenobarbitone which does not need to be in the doctor's handwriting). Doses are written as g, mg, micrograms, 5 ml or 10 ml, and amounts usually as multiples of 50 ml or 25 g. Avoid fractions of a gram or milligram and use the next smaller unit, e.g. write 500 micrograms and not 0.5 mg.

Controlled drugs are controlled by the *Misuse of Drugs Acts* 1971 and 1973. They are graded according to their harmfulness and the penalties for misuse, and include:

Class A: diamorphine*, cocaine*, dipipanone* (Diconal), morphine, pethidine, LSD, methadone (Physeptone), opium, dextromoramide (Palfium) and Class B drugs when injected. Those marked * can only be prescribed by specially licensed doctors when used for patients addicted to them.

Class B: amphetamines, barbiturates, cannabis, codeine, pholcodeine and pentazocine (Fortral).

Class C: diethylpropion (Apisate).

A doctor must *notify the Chief Medical Officer*, Drugs Branch,

Queen Ann's Gate, SW1H 9AT of anyone who seems to be addicted to:

cocaine	dextromoramide (Palfium)
diamorphine (Heroin)	dipipanone (Diconal)
methadone (Physeptone)	morphine
opium	pethidine
hydrocodone	hydromorphine
phenazocine (Narphen)	levorphanol

This does not only apply to patients for whom the doctor is prescribing but also to those suspected of addiction. The notification should be confirmed for each patient annually. Notification should state the patient's name and address, sex, date of birth, NHS number, date of attendance and the names of the drugs to which the patient is suspected of being addicted and whether any prescription was given.

Patients registering as 'temporary residents' and asking for addictive drugs should be treated with caution – check by telephoning their permanent doctor whether the drug requested is genuinely needed.

(5) Suspected *adverse reactions* should be reported to the *Committee on Safety of Medicines* by means of the Yellow Cards provided or by telephone to Freephone Committee on Safety of Medicines. Only serious adverse reactions (i.e. anything that interferes with the patient's normal activities) should be reported and not well known minor reactions, except in the case of new drugs (marked ▼ in the BNF and MIMS) when all adverse reactions should be reported.

(6) Prescription charges did not exceed 20p per item from the beginning of the NHS in 1948 until 1979. From then, they have been gradually increased and were £2.60 per item from 1 April 1988. In 1968, *exemptions* were introduced and since the rapid increase in prescription charges in 1979 the proportion who pay these has gradually reduced from about one third to 18% in July 1986. The following categories of patients are exempt:

- those aged under 16 or over pensionable age – 60 or 65 years
- women who are pregnant or have given birth within the last year
- patients requiring treatment of war disablement
- person drawing Family Credit or Income Support Benefit

(previously Family Income Supplement and Supplementary Benefit before the changes in Social Security regulations in April 1988)

- person whose net income is not more than £1.50 plus the cost of a prescription (total £3.90 in 1987) above that which would entitle them to Supplementary Benefit/Income Support
- person with one of the following conditions:
    venereal disease
    permanent fistula requiring continuous dressing or an appliance (e.g. colostomy)
    diabetes
    hypoparathyroidism, hypothyroidism, hypopituitarism, hypo-adrenalism
    epilepsy
    permanent physical disability preventing the person from moving outside the home without help

Oral contraceptives taken for contraceptive purposes are also free of charge.

(7) It is useful to have a way of adjusting doses quickly in accordance with the patient's age – rather than calculating the dose exactly in relationship to weight and surface area as is necessary for some drugs, e.g. those used for chemotherapy of malignant disease. The following rough method can be used in most cases:

Age	Fraction of adult dosage
Newborn (full term)	1/8
1 year	1/4
3 years	1/3
7 years	1/2
12 years	3/4

(8) Always write full details of drugs in *referral letters* to hospitals. When sharing the care of patients for particular conditions with hospital doctors, it is the doctor with clinical responsibility for the condition being treated who should be responsible for prescribing. In correspondence with the general practitioner, the hospital doctor should make it clear when he or she is passing the clinical and prescribing responsibility back to the general practitioner. This helps to avoid confusion and possible inconvenience or danger to patients. Patients on warfarin, steroids or monoamine oxidase inhibitors, and preferably also those with chronic

conditions such as diabetics, should carry cards showing their drugs and dosages.

(9) Districts and regions have *drug information services* and these can be quite helpful (telephone numbers for the regions may be found in the BNF).

(10) Where possible, prescribe *generically*. The Drug and Therapeutics Bulletin for 30 November 1987 summarized the advantages and disadvantages of generic (approved or non-proprietary) prescribing as follows:

Advantages of generic prescribing

(a) Generic names indicate the chemical class of the drug (e.g. diazepam, lorazepam, nitrazepam and oxazepam are all benzodiazepines).

(b) It helps to avoid confusion for patients, doctors and nurses if the same name is always used for a drug. Generally speaking, generic names are standard throughout the world whereas the brand names vary with each country.

(c) In teaching student nurses and doctors the generic names are used and it is illogical for the student to have to change to brand names.

(d) By law, brand names must be dispensed if they are prescribed. Hence, the use of generic names would permit chemists to reduce the number of named variants of a particular drug that they need to stock and possibly reduce delays if particular brand names are not in stock.

(e) Generic prescribing would probably lead to lower drug costs for the NHS.

Disadvantages of generic prescribing

(a) Brand names are often simpler to write and remember.

(b) Branded and generic drug suppliers must obtain a product licence from the licensing authority before a drug can be marketed and the manufacturer must have a manufacturer's licence. This ensures that drugs are of good quality and of specified bioavailability. Occasionally, unlicensed products can be illegally imported and sold, but this is a criminal offence.

(c) Excipients and colourants are meant to be inert and harmless but there could be differences between branded and generic equivalents which might cause problems in some patients. Occasionally, the different appearance of branded and generic drugs may upset some patients if they are used to a particular brand.

(d) The source of a generic drug may not be identifiable once it has been dispensed, and a patient who suffers from a side-effect may then sue the doctor or pharmacist if the company cannot be identified.

(11) A few general clinical prescribing rules are given below:

(a) Although it may seem obvious, it is a good rule to remember to use medicines only if they are absolutely necessary. Listening to the patient can often be far more helpful than prescribing a drug.

(b) Consciously try to avoid any temptation to use the prescription merely as a means of bringing the consultation to an end.

(c) It is essential to give clear explanations of why, how and for how long to take the drugs, and what to look out for in the way of possible side-effects. For elderly patients, it may be helpful to use a box in which a week's drugs can be laid out in the correct order by a relative or the district nurse.

(d) Use a small number of drugs, preferably from a selected list and by generic name, and get to know them well. Be very cautious about using drugs which have been newly introduced onto the market – particularly in the classes which may have severe side-effects, such as non-steroidal anti-inflammatory drugs.

(e) Use lower dosages in those with poorer renal or liver function – this includes the elderly in general – and try to avoid drugs in pregnancy completely. The BNF gives further details when it is essential to use drugs in any of these circumstances.

(f) Once or twice a day dosages are easier for patients to remember and should be chosen, all other things being equal.

9

The Holistic Approach: Self-care and Complementary Medicine

CRITIQUE OF MODERN MEDICINE ● SYSTEMS THEORY: THE BIO-PSYCHOSOCIAL MODEL ● THE HOLISTIC APPROACH ● ALTERNATIVE/COMPLEMENTARY MEDICINE ● PREVENTIVE AND PROMOTIONAL HEALTH CARE

Many of the advances in thinking that have developed in the context of primary health care have involved exploring and examining areas of medical practice which have, for the most part, been neglected in medical schools and have usually been labelled 'fringe'. Changing public expectations and attitudes, together with an increasing emphasis by the medical profession on the *promotion of health* and the *prevention of disease*, has led to a re-examination of much that has been neglected.

CRITIQUE OF MODERN MEDICINE

The underlying assumptions that have largely governed the way medicine is practised have been based on the *bio-medical* model of human functioning. This model assumes a form of *dualism* that separates the functioning of the mind and body; it leads to a *mechanistic* view of the body and supports a *reductionistic* (reducing things to their smallest parts) approach to the study of disease. Whereas this model has led to enormous advances in pharmacology, surgery and 'high-tech' medicine, it has tended at times to impoverish the more humane aspects of a doctor's role. In recent years, there has been an increasing number of well reasoned arguments concerning the limitations of this approach.

Ivan Illich (who has combined the roles of parish priest in an Irish-Puerto Rican neighbourhood with that of a theologian, social thinker and agent provocateur of many professions) rocked the medical world with his book *Limits to Medicine*, or *Medical Nemesis* as it was first titled in 1976. His principle statement was that 'the medical establishment has become a major threat to health.' He outlined the epidemics of modern medicine and collected a large body of evidence to show how much of modern medical treatment is *useless* and potentially *harmful*. Amongst the many indictments were:

(1) that 15% of all hospital admissions are the result of medically-induced disease
(2) that 7% of all hospital admissions result in some compensatable injury.

Illich then proceeded to illustrate how the medical profession has influenced the health policies of various countries and has developed a stranglehold on *how money is spent on health care and, more importantly,* **where** *it is spent.* He pointed out that because the medical profession is concerned with high technology and the scientific approach, a disproportionate part of our budget is spent on hospital-oriented services to the detriment of basic general practice and community services. The development of coronary care units and expenditure on high cost machines, such as 'scans' and linear accelerators, are a direct result of the medical profession's interests rather than because they benefit the patient.

Illich's most pungent criticisms against the medical profession, however, were levelled at the way it has influenced the belief-systems and values of the patients. He felt that the 'promise' to end all pain and eliminate disease is a massive and tragic dehumanizing confidence trick. Death can never be cheated and the medical profession's attempts to prolong life at all cost robs man of his essential human existence. Illich saw the *medicalization* of many of life's processes – birth, pregnancy, marriage, divorce, death – as an essentially anti-human act and put much of the blame on the medical profession's narrow and limited approach.

Illich's book was largely castigated in the medical press and his arguments, because they appeared so general and one-sided, were not taken too seriously. He failed to see how his case against the medical profession could not be separated from the ideology, culture and the society from which the medical profession arose. The *collusion* so apparent between doctors and patients was not sufficiently touched on, and doctors were made the scapegoats for much that is wrong within their culture. It is important to understand how this 'collusion' prevents both doctor and patient from assuming their full potential. Achieving this potential involves an awareness of both the strengths and limitations present in each role. The doctor's ability to heal is influenced by the extent to which he is aware of the 'patient' within him; and the patient's ability to improve and get better is influenced by the extent to which he is aware of the 'doctor' within him. What has happened in our culture is that all the 'healing powers' have been lodged in the doctor.

In *The Role of Medicine* (1979), Thomas McKeown distanced himself from many of the doctor-bashing remarks in *The Limits to Medicine* and he says 'the two books have little in common except perhaps in the sense that the Bible and the Koran could be said to be identified by the fact that both are concerned with religious matters.' His own approach was to illustrate how 'for most diseases, prevention by control of their origins is cheaper, more humane, and more effective than intervention by treatment after they occur.'

McKeown used a *cultural, social* and *epidemiological* 'pair of spectacles' to look at health and illness in our society. His views have been shared by many of the foremost social explorers of the nineteenth and twentieth century. Many of these reformers went to the very heart of the social and political divisions of our time. Class division, urban poverty and inequality in education all play a part in determining the frequency and type of illness to which individuals are prone. Childbirth is a far more risky event for working-class women than for middle-class women. More recently, the *Black Report* (1982) has highlighted these inequalities in health in our own time.

Ian Kennedy, in his book *The Unmasking of Medicine* (1981), described some of the myths and fancies surrounding how medical decisions, both clinical and political, are made. He used an *ethical, legal* and *philosophical* 'pair of spectacles' to look at the relationship between doctor and patient as well as medicine and society, and has drawn attention to the political nature of decisions surrounding the purchase of kidney machines, old people's homes and drug expenditure.

SYSTEMS THEORY: THE BIO-PSYCHOSOCIAL MODEL

Systems theory has received prominence through the writings of Weiss and Von Bertalanffy, but it was George Engel who applied this model to health and illness. Engel used the model table to study human *functioning*. He saw man as functioning within a hierarchy of natural systems – a system being defined as an 'organized dynamic whole' having sufficient persistence and identity to justify being so named.

Engel pointed out how each system is at the same time a component of higher systems, i.e. a cell is part of tissue and tissue forms part of an organ and so on. Nothing exists in isolation – no man is an island – but each system carries its own uniqueness and thus calls for its own method of study and ultimately develops its own language. General systems theory attempts to explain the laws governing the interaction between systems and makes links between the biological sciences and social sciences.

The *bio-psychosocial model* has gone some way to answer the limitations of the bio-medical model. The following brief example might illustrate how this model can enlarge and inform the *diagnostic process*, as well as expand the notion of treatment.

> A 27-year old Spaniard presented with the classical symptoms of duodenal ulcer subsequently proved on x-ray. He had left his native country after a troubled affair with his partner's wife and was unsettled and out of work in London. He was a practising Catholic and was much troubled by his affair. He was eating sporadically and drinking heavily.

Using the model in Figure 9.1 one can develop an understanding of this man's illness depending on which 'level' or sub-system one explores, e.g.

'Cause'	*Level*	*Treatment*
Poor housing		Social intervention
Unemployment	Society	
Marital disharmony	Family	Marriage guidance
Excess stress		Relaxation Diet Counselling

Stomach dysfunction	Organ	Vagotomy
Erosion of gastric mucosa	Tissue	Barrier e.g. carbenoxolene
Excess acid production	Cell	Antacids
H_2 receptor	Molecule	H_2 antagonist

No one sub-system is 'right' but allowing for more than one view will allow for a broader and holistic model to emerge.

THE HOLISTIC APPROACH

The word 'holism' was first used by Smuts in 1928 in his book *Holism and Evolution* and is derived from the Greek meaning whole or complete. Smuts used the word 'holistic' to describe the philosophical systems that looked on *whole* systems rather than parts. It is unfortunate that the word holistic has been linked with 'alternative medicine' for the term is not about a method of treatment but about an approach. *The holistic approach to health and disease is equally found amongst orthodox medical practitioners as amongst alternative practitioners.* The following four basic principles govern the holistic approach:

(1) *The whole is greater than the sum of its parts*

It is necessary when examining a diseased or malfunctioning *part* to look at and be aware of the *whole* (person, family etc.). Focusing and 'treating' the whole may restore the functioning of the part. The application of this principle has been outlined above and draws heavily on systems theory.

(2) *The use of a wide range of medical interventions*

Orthodox medicine has often limited itself to the belief that healing requires mainly drugs or surgery. It is very quickly apparent to most general practitioners that often the best 'alternative medicine' is to listen to the patient. Yet very few doctors have had any thorough training in communication skills. The holistic approach espouses the use of:

(a) *Orthodox approaches* – drugs, surgery, radiotherapy

(b) *Communication 'therapies'* – listening, counselling advice, psychotherapy

(c) *Self-help skills* – breathing and relaxation, meditation, physical exercise, dietary counselling

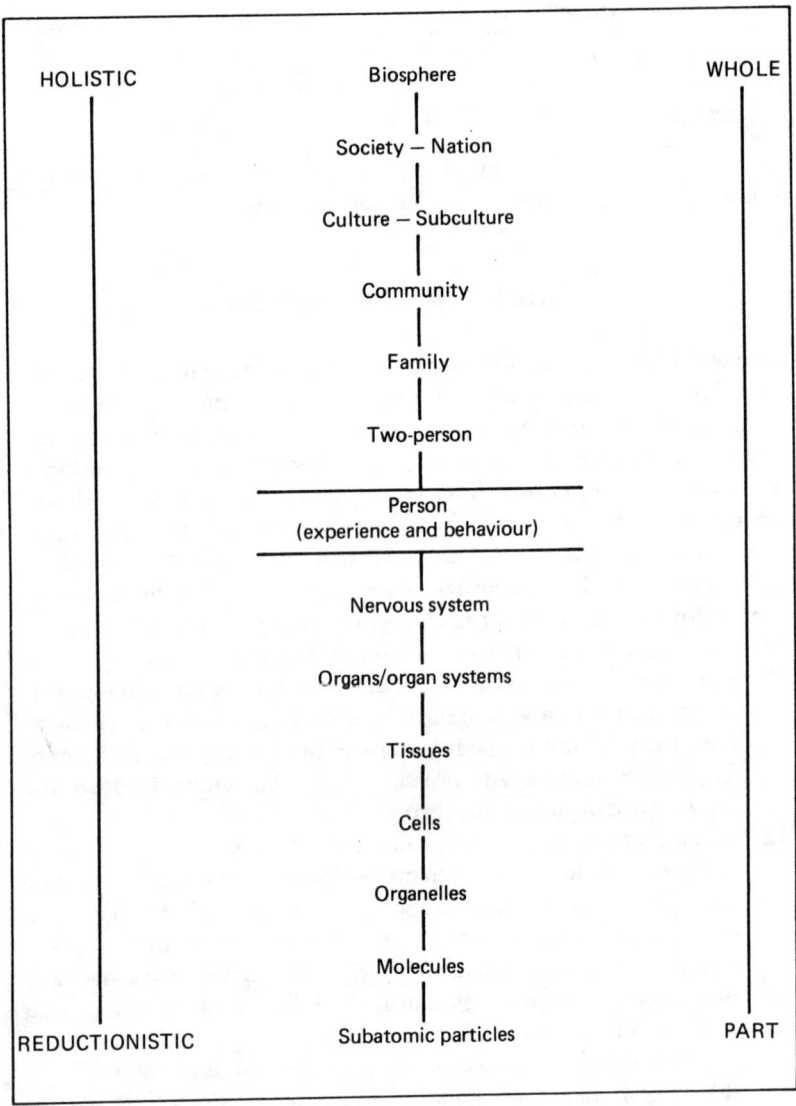

Figure 9.1 The hierarchy of natural systems (from Engel 1980).

(d) *Alternative or complementary therapies* – acupuncture, herbal medicine, osteopathy, homoeopathy, chiropractic etc.

It is the inclusion of the latter two categories (expanded below) that is more often than not incorrectly identified as being 'the holistic approach'.

(3) *Responsibility and health care*

One of the main foci in a holistic approach is to encourage and nurture the patient's own homoeostatic-regulatory mechanism (*self-healing*). This requires a shift for both doctors and patients: the doctor to let go of his need to 'cure' the patient, and the patient to let go of his wish to be treated like a passive participant and to assume some responsibility for his health. This shift towards a more participatory relationship is of necessity a relative one as there will always be legitimate reasons for a doctor to assume an active curative role, e.g. accidents or surgical intervention. However, it is increasingly clear that many of the problems seen in general practice are related to life-style, work routines, interpersonal relationships and health beliefs. In addition, many of the chronic 'incurable' conditions – arthritis, diabetes, cancer, heart disease – require a move from a 'curative' to a caring approach. Encouraging patients to assume greater responsibility for their health care is not easy and can be fraught with danger. It is unnecessary and cruel to increase a patient's distress by increasing his 'guilt' concerning the causation of his illness. (This issue will be enlarged upon in the section on self-care.) The shift in role necessitates a shift in how doctors engage with patients. The *unit of medical exchange* has been the individual consultation; moving from a curing to an educational role may involve seeing patients in groups and in a classroom setting. Patients can be given basic health information as well as taught simple 'coping skills' to enable them to look after themselves more effectively.

(4) *Physician heal thyself*

There is an increasing number of studies concerned with the level of morbidity and mortality amongst *doctors*. These studies indicate a greater than expected rate of depression, divorce, drug abuse and suicide. The effect that this level of illness amongst doctors has on their ability to care for others is not as yet sufficiently understood. Nevertheless, it must be of increasing concern even if only because of the toll on the medical profession. Similar concerns have been expressed regarding the health of nurses and social workers, and suggestions for change have involved a thorough reappraisal of the undergraduate curriculum.

The medical school years are divided into pre-clinical and clinical years. Unfortunately, they may also become the *pre-cynical* and *cynical* years. Medical students arrive at medical schools with some sense of hope, concern, compassion and idealism as befits many nineteen-year olds. As they struggle with the enormous amount of information required to pass exams, they begin to have some of their idealism blunted by the many hours of hard work involved. When they eventually go on the wards, they meet patients who are ill, but also who are anxious, frightened, depressed, angry and, at times, rude and difficult. They see patients in pain and in tears, and witness the last breath of a human being as he struggles for his life.

The instruction and guidance that students are given on how to handle these difficult human situations are often not sufficient. Rather, they are asked about the state of the patient's liver or the latest blood test. There is no doubt that this sort of instruction is essential – the high technical competence of our doctors is proof enough of that – but what is the cost of concentrating so much on these aspects? As the students struggle, not only with having to amass a new set of knowledge, they are overwhelmed with feelings they do not understand. Even worse, they may stop feeling altogether as a protection from these difficulties.

Nearly 50% of medical students eventually enter general practice. It is a common observation that the process of becoming a qualified general practitioner involves 'unlearning' many of the assumptions, behaviour and skills picked up at medical school. Much of general practice postgraduate education requires the individual to broaden his thinking and adopt a more holistic approach to the problems presented to him. This involves what Balint described as a 'limited though considerable change in the doctor's personality.' It may be that unless he understands this change, the future doctor will be more liable to suffer from the stresses and strain of his demanding occupation.

ALTERNATIVE/COMPLEMENTARY MEDICINE

More than one million people a year seek the help of alternative practitioners. It is estimated there are more than 30 000 alternative practitioners in the UK (more than the number of general practitioners), and that one in seven of the population has, at some time or another, consulted such a practitioner. Some of these practitioners have had no training, whereas others have attended rigorous full-time courses in some ways comparable to the undergraduate curriculum. It is not surprising, then, if there is confusion about what alternative/complementary medicine is and whether it has anything to offer at the level of primary care. Several surveys have indicated the increasing interest and use of alternative therapies by general practitioners. Amongst 100 general practitioner trainees, a positive attitude emerged in 86, and 70 expressed a wish to undergo training in one or more of these therapies. Of 145 general practitioners responding to a postal questionnaire, 55 (38%) had received some training, and 22 (15%) wished to arrange training.

The term *alternative medicine* is used to describe those therapies and approaches to healing that are not covered by the traditional medical undergraduate curriculum. The word *complementary* is used by some as a way of avoiding the confrontational aspect with traditional medicine. It is helpful to separate the numerous different approaches into the following groups:

Group I Complete system of healing (having a theoretical, diagnostic, investigative and therapeutic understanding of health and disease)
(1) acupuncture
(2) herbal medicine
(3) osteopathy
(4) chiropractic
(5) homoeopathy.

Group II Diagnostic methods
(1) kinesiology
(2) iridology
(3) hair analysis
(4) aura diagnosis.

Group III Therapeutic modalities
(1) massage
(2) reflexology
(3) aromatherapy
(4) spirituality.

Group IV Self-help measures
(1) breathing and relaxation
(2) meditation

(3) exercise

(4) diet therapy.

The most common types of practitioner consulted by the public are in the first group (see Table 9.1), although it is clear that participation in self-help measures is increasing and many practitioners will include advice on self-help as part of their therapeutic approach. The British Medical Association (BMA) *Report on Complementary Therapies* attempts to provide some objective guide to the efficacy and suitability of alternative methods of health care.

Table 9.1 *Most common types of complementary practitioners consulted by the public*

Osteopathy	42%
Homoeopathy	26%
Acupuncture	23%
Chiropractic	22%
Herbalism	11%

The *British Holistic Medical Association* considered that the BMA report was faulty and misconceived, and did not help the current confusion. Nevertheless, the BMA report identified several factors which were felt to be significant and possibly explained the popularity of alternative medicine. These were the *amount of time* available to the patient, the use of *touch* (common to many alternative therapies), and the *magical* quality surrounding some of the practitioners and their therapies. For the scientific doctor trained in critical evaluation, it is important that the issue of the efficacy of these therapies is addressed. Although substantial research studies exist for Group IV (self-help measures), the paucity of good clinical studies has hampered the acceptance of Group I (complementary systems of healing). Similarly, the lack of any clear training and regulatory standards amongst the complementary practitioners has led to the term *fringe medicine*. It is important for doctors to avoid the error of dismissing as unfounded what may in fact be both true and important, whilst rightly insisting on avoiding the error of accepting as true what has not been proved.

Five major complementary therapies which offer good training, and have regulatory bodies with ethical and clinical guidelines, will be briefly described:

Acupuncture

This is an approach to treatment based on the Chinese model of health and disease. In this model, it is felt that in addition to a circulatory and nervous system, *energy* flows in channels called *meridians* and disease occurs where the energy flow is blocked for whatever reason. Needles are placed in different parts of the body which help to 'unblock' energy channels. The placing of needles is only one aspect of acupuncture; a physician trained in traditional Chinese medicines will take a very long time to arrive at his 'diagnosis' and will pay particular attention to diet, emotional factors and environmental aspects.

In England, there are two 'schools' of acupuncture practice. One is based on the traditional Chinese approach, is practised mostly by non-doctors and generally accepts a wide range of problems. The second school is practised by doctors and is based much more on a western model of disease; acupuncture (the placing of needles) is seen as an additional 'treatment' and is most commonly utilized for muscular and arthritic conditions – the relief of pain and occasionally for anaesthesia.

Recent neurophysiological experiments have led to an understanding of how acupuncture works in language that is derived from western scientific thinking. The most recent has involved the relationship between the use of acupuncture and *endorphin* release. Several studies have demonstrated that the effects of acupuncture and trans-electrical nerve stimulation (TENS) are mediated through the release of endorphins and naloxone – a morphine antagonist – may reverse effects, although the evidence is still not conclusive. The endorphin-acupuncture link, although persuasive, may not be the total explanation as other neurotransmitters (e.g. 5-hydroxytryptamine) appear to be released as well.

Osteopathy

This is a well accepted approach for the treatment of many muscular, skeletal and arthritic conditions. The practitioners receive good training and treat these conditions with a combination of *massage*, *manipulation*, *exercise* retraining and *postural* advice. Quite often a low back pain, not managed by conventional medical treatment (drugs, rest or surgery), has been dramatically helped by the use of osteopathic techniques. Some osteopaths expand their clinical practice to include more general conditions, e.g. asthma and migraine, and their 'success' may be more a reflection of their own caring personalities than the therapy itself.

Chiropractic

This is very similar to osteopathy but is much less available in the UK. The difference between osteopathy and chiropractic has more to do with the type of manipulative technique used and the range of conditions treated.

Homoeopathy

This branch of complementary medicine has a long and traditional history in Britain, having been the preferred approach to treatment amongst many members of the Royal family. The majority of homoeopaths are doctors who have been trained in a conventional manner. Homoeopathy is a system of treatments which use *remedies* rather than drugs. These remedies contain minute levels of extracts which have no 'chemical effect' on the body. Homoeopaths believe remedies work as a result of the fundamental principle of homoeopathy that *like cures like*. By this it is meant that, rather than suppress or destroy a symptom or infection (as modern drugs do), cure is achieved by stimulating the body's own healing powers. This is done by giving a remedy which, in much greater doses, would *produce* the actual symptom about which the patient is complaining. There is no doubt that homoeopathy is a safe method of treatment and that in several conditions it appears to have a dramatic effect. Conventional doctors are still unconvinced that it has a part to play in the treatment of disease, however, and there has been little objective evidence to indicate that homoeopathy is effective in acute and chronic disease states. Nevertheless, for many of the minor to moderately severe non-life-threatening conditions, homoeopathy appears to be safe. It must be pointed out that many of these conditions are self-limiting and would probably improve whatever therapy was used.

Herbal medicine

There is a long tradition of using herbs for the treatment of medical conditions – indeed, many of our most effective drugs are derived from medical herbs, e.g. digoxin (foxglove). Herbalists are trained in anatomy, physiology and diagnosis much like most doctors, but instead of drugs use herbs for their therapies. Herbalists will treat the whole gamut of medical conditions although they will be quite happy to refer back to the doctor those conditions which are better treated by conventional means.

About 100 herbal products are estimated to be on the market and very few people actually consult a herbalist before purchasing these products. The majority are available from health-food shops and pharmacists. Concern has been expressed as to their safety as well as their efficacy, and currently the *Committee on the Review of Medicines* is undertaking an examination of these products.

PREVENTIVE AND PROMOTIONAL HEALTH CARE

The increasing focus on preventive and promotional health care suggests that studies to assess the value of self-care may well be one direction in which general practice research should go.

In 1976, a series of official reports published by the DHSS brought the whole theme of prevention into new prominence. Shortly afterwards, the Royal College of General Practitioners published a series of reports on specific areas of preventive work in general practice – psychiatric disorders, family planning, arterial disease and child health. In these reports, *anticipatory care* – the union of prevention of disease and the promotion of health with care and cure – is proposed as the main direction of the primary medical services in the foreseeable future.

Prevention means removing the risks that disease will occur by programmes of immunization, halting the consequences of established disease by early detection and treatment, and promoting health by helping people to learn and accept responsibility for their own well-being. This emphasis on anticipatory care also implies a growing desire to view health and the practice of medicine from a broader conceptual and clinical base than primarily as pathology correction and specialist treatment. With the mushrooming of the related specialties of behavioural medicine, psychophysiology, health psychology and psychoneuroimmunology, there is some experimental evidence that emotion and behaviour are intimately bound up with the central nervous system processes governing autonomic, endocrine and immunological activity. Indeed, many authors feel that medical conditions that are 'stress-induced' have long since replaced epidemics of infectious disease as some of the major medical problems. The four most common conditions – cardiovascular, cancer, arthritis and respiratory diseases – are increasingly being related to problems with life-style, i.e. diet and nutrition, environmental factors and psychosocial stress.

Self-care

There has been a surge of public interest in recent years in self-care and self-help therapies. Levin described self-care as 'those activities individuals undertake in promoting their own health, preventing their own disease, limiting their own illness and restoring their own health.' John Fry identified four roles for self-care – self-diagnosis, self-treatment, disease prevention and health maintenance – and we shall briefly outline each of these categories.

(1) *Self-diagnosis* The majority of the population on developing a symptom will attempt to make sense of it according to their level of knowledge and understanding. Over 88% of patients seek advice from friends and family before consulting a general practitioner. Other sources of information include books, 'phone-ins and agony aunts, and 3.5% of patients tap at least five different sources before going to the doctor.

One of the forces promoting self-care amongst the public has been the wish to develop more autonomy and to de-medicalize certain 'normal' life situations. This is clearly seen in the area of the *women's health movement* and the purchase of home sphygomanometers. Nevertheless, a difficulty in developing a rational policy towards self-diagnosis and self-treatment, especially of minor complaints, is the problem of agreement amongst professionals as to what constitutes a minor symptom— i.e. one not requiring medical attention. A research study to evaluate a policy of self-care had to be abandoned because the participants, all experienced general practitioners, could not agree amongst themselves.

Self-diagnosis need not imply a medical knowledge of complex physiological processes, but can include a form of self-monitoring ranging from height and weight measurement to breast examination and urine testing. The latter two procedures initially require instruction but need not involve any medical person.

(2) *Self-treatment* Almost always this implies a form of self-medication. Over one third of the total drug bill is from over-the-counter sales and, at any one time, two thirds of the population have taken self-prescribed medication in the preceeding fortnight. The medicines most commonly consumed without a prescription are outlined in Table 9.2.

Table 9.2 *Medicines consumed by categories and the proportion of these in NHS prescriptions*

Therapeutic group	Proportion of people taking medicine in a fortnight		NHS prescriptions
	(1)	(2)	(3)
Analgesics	38	41	7
Skin preparations	20	14	7
Antacids etc.	12	14	5
Cough medicines	18	13	10
Sedatives etc.	4	10	17
Laxatives	9	9	3
Tonics etc.	22	19	6

Sources: (1) Wadsworth et al. (1971); (2) Dunnell and Cartwright (1972); (3) Office of Population Censuses and Surveys, *et al.* (1973).

General practitioners' evaluations of patients' self-treatment is largely positive – only 5% of self-medication is thought to be potentially harmful. This must be contrasted with the potentially very real harmful effects of prescribed drugs. Nevertheless, professional concern at the over-use of non-prescribed medication is real and appropriate.

Other forms of treatment adopted by the public before, after or instead of consulting the doctor, include traditional folk remedies, charms (e.g. a copper bracelet for rheumatism), visits to spas, faith healers and the whole gamut of alternative and complementary medicines described above. A major development in this field has been the growth of *self-help groups*. Several distinct types of such groups exist, some providing information only, some acting as support groups providing assistance and help, and some initiating research into forms of treatment not available through orthodox channels.

(3) *Disease prevention* Traditionally, this has been the area of health education and doctor-led activities (see Chapter 4 *Epidemiology and Prevention in General Practice*, p. 59). *Primary prevention* is aimed at avoiding the disease altogether e.g. immunization or anti-smoking campaigns. *Secondary prevention* involves catching the disease at an early stage, e.g. cervical screening or mammography, and *tertiary prevention* involves limiting the effect of a disease once the patient has developed it, e.g. diabetic monitoring. All these preventive activities still necessitate expert care and advice but rely on the cooperation and motivation of the patient. Some can be seen to rely solely on patient participation and are individually based – others may form part of social policy and require political action, e.g. fluoridation, food policies on additives, Clean Air Acts etc.

Screening as a form of disease prevention has attracted much attention but the initial enthusiasm has been tempered by a realization of the limitation of any mass programme which is not accompanied by an emphasis on health behaviour. The World Health Organization, in an attempt to help health administration develop a rational policy towards screening, outlined the following ten basic questions:

- Is the natural history of the disease fully known?
- Is the disease significant (a common and/or serious health problem)?
- Is there a recognizable latent or presymptomatic stage?
- Is there a reliable screening test?
- Are the facilities for full elucidation and treatment of detected abnormalities available?
- Is there an agreed treatment for the disease?
- Can screening be carried out as a continuing process?
- Is there agreement on the groups of people at risk from the disease?
- Is the screening test acceptable to the people to be screened?
- Is the cost-effectiveness of screening better than that of previous practice?

(4) *Health maintenance* There has been a welcome interest in the pursuit of a 'healthy life-style' as a counterbalance to the search for the magic bullet. Attendance at jogging clubs, meditation groups,

relaxation classes and health food stores increase yearly. There have been several attempts to introduce such activities into general practice but, as yet, no long-term research to indicate the benefit of this approach to health maintenance.

Belloc, in one of the few studies, followed 7000 adults for more than five years and identified those behaviours that were thought to affect health. Mortality at all ages was influenced by *way of life*, especially hours of sleep, regularity of meals, weight, smoking and drinking. Other short term studies have indicated the benefit of *respiratory retraining* and muscular relaxation in the hyperventilation syndrome, hypertension, postoperative analgesia requirements and migraine.

Meditation can be described as a practice which induces a state of non-physiological arousal, and several studies have indicated both the immediate physiological changes (fall in pulse rate, reduction in respiratory rate, increase in brainwave activity) as well as the clinical benefits in anxiety/depression, hypertension and insomnia.

The pursuit of such practices requires a motivation which may not always be present, yet it is clearly possible to introduce this form of 'health maintenance' into general practice. A recent study in a North London Health Centre demonstrated both short-term and long-term (one year) effects of introducing such an approach. Nevertheless, more research needs to be carried out before the medical profession accepts these activities as a legitimate addition to their work in primary health centres.

The climate of opinion has altered substantially in the last ten years. Several meetings between orthodox and complementary practitioners have occurred to discuss issues on training, research and referral procedures. The General Medical Council has eased its regulations concerning referral, and more and more general practitioners are involved in direct work with complementary practitioners in addition to seeking additional training themselves.

REFERENCES AND FURTHER READING

Dunnell K., Cartwright A. (1972). *Medicine Takers, Prescribers and Hoarders*. London: Routledge & Kegan Paul.

Engel G. (1980). The clinical application of the bio-psychosocial model. *Am. J. Psych.*, **137**, 535.

Illich I. (1976). *Limits to Medicine*. London: Marion Boyars Publishers.

McKeown T. (1979). *The Role of Medicine – Dream, Mirage or Nemesis?* Oxford: Basil Blackwell.

Office of Population Censuses and Surveys, Department of Health and Social Security, Royal College of General Practitioners (1973). *Morbidity Statistics from General Practice – Second National Study*. Studies in Medical and Population Subjects No. 26. London: HMSO.

Pietroni P. C., McLean J., Walton N. G. (1987). Introducing a self-care programme into general practice. *Practitioner*, **231**, 1226.

Smuts J. C. (1926). *Holism and Evolution*. New York: Macmillan Publishing Company.

Wadsworth M. E. J., Blamey R., Butterfield W. J. H. (1971). *Health and Sickness: the Choice of Treatment*. London: Tavistock Publications.

Primary Health Care In Developing Countries

**THE PHILOSOPHY OF PRIMARY HEALTH CARE ● PRACTICAL
ASPECTS OF PRIMARY HEALTH CARE ● EXAMPLES OF
PRIMARY CARE SYSTEMS ● PRIMARY HEALTH CARE
PERSONNEL ● MATERNAL AND CHILD HEALTH ● FAMILY
PLANNING ● POLITICAL, PLANNING AND FINANCIAL
CONSIDERATIONS ● SOCIAL AND CULTURAL FACTORS ●
GLOBAL PERSPECTIVE ● THE FUTURE**

The WHO-UNICEF meeting in Alma-Ata in 1978 summarized primary health care as 'essential health care based on practical, scientifically sound and socially acceptable methods and technology, made universally available to individuals and families in the community through their full participation and at a cost that the community and the country can afford to maintain at every stage of their development in the spirit of self-reliance and self-determination'.

In effect, this new found confidence in community-based front line approaches meant that not only a new *method* but a new *philosophy* for providing health care on a mass basis to every section of society was developing.

THE PHILOSOPHY OF PRIMARY HEALTH CARE

Gill Walt and Patrick Vaughan (1981) have emphasized that in 'its original and narrowest sense primary health care means "first contact care" where patients meet health workers. It is the level at which common complaints are treated and preventive measures such as immunizations are carried out.' For developing countries, however, the *Alma-Ata declaration* means that this approach is underlined by five main principles.

(1) *Equitable distribution of health care resources* Health services must be equally accessible in all areas, not neglecting for example rural isolated populations or peri-urban dwellers.

(2) *Community involvement and participation* Active and continuous participation by the community in their own health decisions is essential.

(3) *Focus on prevention* Preventive and promotive services, as well as curative services, should be the focus of health care.

(4) *Use of appropriate technology* The materials and methods used in the health system should be acceptable and relevant – appropriate technology not being synonymous with primitive or poor technology.

(5) *Adoption of a multi-sectoral approach* Health must be seen as part of total care – nutrition, education, water supplies and shelter are all essential minimum requirements to well-being.

Thus, a focus on primary health care in developing countries must concentrate on accessible, innovative and flexible systems which operate within a wide variety of settings and under a variety of political, economic and social frameworks. Primary health care therefore refers to a *level* of health care and to a *set of activities* performed at the point of contact between the health system and the community. Existing systems may firstly be underfinanced and secondly provide inadequate coverage of all sections of the population. The subsequent importance of *community health workers*, who form an integral part of good quality primary care in the developing world through 'low cost' community health care programmes or using simple health activities, has often given rise to the erroneous view that it is second-rate medicine for the lower social classes. This is of course untrue: primary health care systems provide suitable standards of preventive and curative practice outside the framework of hospitals and sophisticated technology in order to meet the priority needs of all sectors of the population.

The *financial* implications of primary health care services have to be considered within the overall economic framework. Developed countries devote 5–10% of their gross national product to direct health service expenditure. Some underdeveloped countries today devote no more than 2% of their much smaller gross national products to health services. Current annual per capita expenditure on health in the developing world is about US$11 compared with an average of US$320 in developed nations.

Health care needs are usually best catered for by localized *small scale* health services appropriate to the communities they serve. However, hospital services based on western curative health care models are often seen by developing, and indeed developed, countries to answer their immediate health care problems. In the Third World, such projects are very costly and swallow up a large portion of public and private spending. They are usually based in urban areas and are highly 'visible' evidence to the population that the government is doing something about the nation's health – contrasting with the less 'visible' small scale village health worker projects in the rural areas.

More importantly, the development of a non-hospital based primary care system built around specific workers in individual communities is cheaper for countries whose national budgets are frequently cut into by debt repayments and military expenditure. In Tanzania, for example, the cost of educating and training one medical graduate was £14 700, for a rural medical assistant £880, and for a rural medical aide £425. So for the price of one qualified doctor, there could be 17 medical assistants and 35 aides. The World Health Organization estimates that on average, for the cost of training one doctor a country could get five nurses, 24 medical assistants and 50 sanitary inspectors (Sanders, 1985).

In addition to this, the primary health care philosophy implies that good primary care in the community leads to a more efficient use of hospital services. In a study of under-fives in hospital in the capital of Cameroon it was concluded that 'our problem in Yaounde did not lie in an inability to treat effectively those children who made it to hospital; it lay in not being able to reach the many who did not come in and in not being able to provide proper care earlier and on a mass basis to the tens of thousands of children with major and minor illnesses in the surrounding community (Joseph, 1985).'

Furthermore, the balance between *curative* and *preventive* care is to a large extent financially determined. 'Expenditure on preventive health care is more easily postponed than expenditure on curative care. The lower a household's or a country's income, the more likely it is that only the most immediate needs are provided for. In the case of health care, curing acute illness obviously represents a more pressing need than reducing latent illness or the risk of future illness' (Zschock, 1979).

Before the Alma-Ata declaration it was often assumed that developing countries were 'as yet unformed infant versions of modern western societies' (Walt and Vaughan 1981). This, combined with the perpetuation of a colonial mentality by the western powers in terms of assessing the developing world's potential and achievements, led to models of social, economic and health care changes being based on western values and philosophies. Coupled with this was the booming movement of inter-governmental aid and development which frequently stressed the overriding importance of investment in the physical elements of national growth – such as dams, roads, power stations – and created or exacerbated the dependence of many Third World countries on western economic and political forces. In addition, 'the need for politicians and governments to produce material proof of their concern for the voting population, the desire of doctors to practise hospital medicine, and the attitudes of health planners and government officials, has meant that commitment to the *'developed' medical model* has been continued in many developing countries' (Liddell, 1985). In effect, primary health care systems for rural areas usually have had to develop alongside hospital medicine for the urban elite. Often, primary health care support systems suffer when funds become short and they must compete with hospitals or other government ministries for financial resources.

Primary health care therefore seeks through localized community participation with both national and local government to establish *appropriate* and *accessible* systems of care for all sections of the population. Services are thus extended to those who are frequently socially or economically marginalized outside the established political structure, such as the rural landless populations, slum dwellers on the edge of large urban conurbations, migrant or seasonal workers, and the disabled or elderly who are expected to be cared for by their families. In practice, this shift in basic approach frequently means favouring groups who have little political or economic influence.

PRACTICAL ASPECTS OF PRIMARY HEALTH CARE

The basic components of an effective primary health care service should be based around the following principles:

(1) *education* about diseases, health problems and their control
(2) *safe water* and basic sanitation
(3) *maternal and child care*, including family planning
(4) *immunization* against major infectious diseases

(5) *appropriate treatment* of common diseases and injuries

(6) provision of *essential drugs*.

It is commonly thought that the most effective, appropriate and economical way of delivering this service is 'through a network of auxiliary health workers and, where practical, traditional practitioners integrated with the health services. A referral network should exist to give mutual support at all levels for patients requiring medical care not available locally' (Sanders, 1985).

The primary health care approach, however, presupposes the existence of a homogeneous community, geographically well defined, open to innovation and new ideas, and with set health needs and requirements – a situation rarely found in reality. The rural/urban dichotomy, together with the frequent polarization of governmental, public and private interests, must also be taken into account. Following the Chinese example, India is trying to place a community health volunteer in all of its 600 000 villages. Yet access to, and the quality of, primary care in peripheral rural villages is often poor, as the nature of the plural society with its class and caste divisions, combined with the mixed economy comprising both public and private sectors, means that underprivileged groups remain underprivileged if the bureaucratic and social structure impedes their access to an already minimal health care system.

No single variable gives an overall indication of the health of an entire community or country but the *infant mortality rate* (IMR – the number of deaths in the first year of life per 1000 live births), together with the measure of *life expectancy* at birth, gives a general impression of mortality trends.

Two factors must, however, be taken into consideration; firstly, the fact that infant mortality rates and other variables are notoriously difficult to collect owing to the under-reporting of births and deaths in many countries, and secondly, differences may exist within selected communities due to social, economic, political or nutritional factors. In South Africa, for example, infant mortality rates in 1970 were roughly six times higher for black and coloured people as they were for whites, whilst in Bangladesh in 1975, a child whose family had no land was five times as likely to die between the ages of one and four years as a child whose family had three acres or more (Sanders, 1985). Indeed, one of the benefits of introducing primary health care services may be that records of morbidity and mortality rates are kept systematically, possibly for the first time.

In parts of Africa and South Asia nearly two thirds of *all* deaths are children under five years old, and in countries where infant and child mortality rates have been reduced, mortality at the ages 1–4 years has fallen first and most rapidly whilst perinatal mortality (deaths from the 28th week of gestation to the seventh day of life per 1000 live and still births) has declined much more slowly.

The key to reducing infant mortality rates within a primary health care framework frequently lies in simple, cost-effective, practical health care techniques which are often linked to broader aspects of social change. In many areas, *tetanus* may account for up to 10% of all neo-natal mortality (deaths in the first month of life) but *diarrhoeal diseases*, closely followed by *respiratory infections*, are the leading cause of morbidity and mortality in the first year of life. *Malnutrition* as an underlying cause (and one which often precipitates the onset of infection and disease) has been cited as responsible for up to 57% of mortality between one month and one year (WHO, 1980).

Simple health prevention techniques that can be implemented at a village or community level under the auspices of a primary care worker can contribute significantly to reducing infant mortality rates. The encouragement of *breast-feeding* for example is an effective measure for the prevention of malnutrition and protection against infection. Evidence from developing countries indicates that infants breast-fed for less than six months or not at all have a mortality 5–10 times higher in the second six months of life than those breast-fed for six months or more. The promotion of milk substitutes by western multinational companies in the developing world can lead to marked increases in infant mortality rates if bottle feeding becomes 'status linked' but cannot be properly carried out and milk powder is mixed incorrectly in unsterile conditions, often with contaminated water.

Breast-feeding, a key concept of the primary health care strategy decided at Alma-Ata, is often difficult to carry out in practice. Save the Children Fund workers in Dacca, Bangladesh, found that: 'Poor mothers may bottle feed for two reasons; one is the example of the rich; the other is the need to work. Women who work as maids of ayahs often have to leave their babies at home. Those who carry out manual labour may know that it is safer not to have the child with them all day. In these circumstances, the only way to feed the infant is to leave a bottle given by an older child or a relative. This malnutrition cannot be blamed on the mother's ignorance alone. It is the result of her poverty, of a lack of facilities for breast-feeding whilst at work and a lack of suitable sheltered employment for destitute women. It is also quite possible that an undernourished anaemic woman cannot produce enough milk to feed her baby. This again is not her fault; it is the result of her poverty. She can be urged to improve her infant feeding practices but she may have severe problems in doing so' (Wheeler and Khanum, 1985).

The *education of women* has also been seen to be a key to better health of the population as a whole. A study by the International Centre for Diarrhoeal Disease Research in Dacca found that better education of any household member (but particularly of mothers) is consistently associated with improved child survival. Educated mothers make earlier and more effective use of health services (Chen, 1986).

Dehydration from diarrhoea kills over four million children each year in developing countries and simple, cheap measures, such as the use of *oral rehydration solution*, can be effective in counteracting this. A solution containing 1.0 g sodium chloride, 1.5 g sodium bicarbonate, 1.5 g potassium chloride and 40 g glucose dissolved in one litre of boiled water, can be used effectively to treat dehydration irrespective of the cause of the diarrhoea which is usually linked to overall social and nutritional status. Severely undernourished children experience on average four times the number of attacks of diarrhoea per year as adequately nourished children. Repeated episodes of diarrhoea impair appetite by making it more difficult for the body to absorb food.

Similarly, simple *immunization* measures have a dramatic impact on reducing childhood mortality. According to the Center for Disease Control in Atlanta, the elimination of immunizable diseases would reduce childhood mortality by 18–35%, and 50% of such deaths would be prevented by the adoption of both oral rehydration combined with basic immunization. Bearing in mind that some 100 million children under the age of five years suffer from protein energy malnutrition, infection by what are seen in the West as routinely preventable childhood diseases can be fatal. The Save the Children Fund reported that during the Ethiopian famine in 1984–5, fatality from measles was up by 50%. Other infectious diseases such as whooping cough and pneumonia begin to appear in the second half of the first year or in the second year of life and, combined with malnutrition, they lead to high mortality rates. Systematic childhood immunization can prevent a number of these illnesses from occurring, but support networks, technical systems such as 'cold chain storage' and transport, and other infrastructural considerations for the delivery of vaccines as well as call-up and recall systems, are often difficult to coordinate. Immunization against diphtheria, tetanus, tuberculosis, measles and polio have also been proven to have significant effects on mortality rates.

Some countries in both the developed and the developing world have, through a variety of political and social changes, made substantial improvements to their infant mortality rates over the years by means of large scale primary care planning encompassing a commitment to health care through small village-based schemes which incorporate some of the ideas mentioned above. The infant mortality rates, together with other variables, of various countries between 1960 and 1985 can be seen in Table 10.1 below:

Table 10.1   *Infant mortality rates (IMR) in 1960 and 1985*

	IMR 1960	IMR 1985	POPN (millions) 1985	GNP (US$ per cap) 1984	Life expectancy (years) 1985
Afghanistan	215	189	16.5	–	38
Mali	210	175	8.1	140	43
Ethiopia	175	152	43.6	110	41
Mozambique	174	147	14.0	230	46
Senegal	180	137	6.4	380	44
Bangladesh	156	124	101.1	130	49
India	165	105	758.9	260	57
Peru	142	94	19.7	1000	60
Nicaragua	140	69	3.2	860	62
China	150	36	1059.5	310	69
Costa Rica	84	19	2.6	1190	73
Cuba	62	15	10.0	–	74
USA	26	11	238.0	15 390	75
UK	23	10	56.1	8570	74
Japan	31	6	120.7	10 630	77
Sweden	16	6	8.4	11 860	76

POPN = population; GNP = gross national product.
Source: UNICEF (1987).

EXAMPLES OF PRIMARY CARE SYSTEMS

Mali

This land-locked country in West Africa has a population of approximately seven million, 16.7% of whom live in urban areas. Like the other Sahel countries surrounding it – Niger, Burkina Faso and Mauritania – Mali suffered greatly during the 1974–5 famine and more recently during the drought from the end of 1984 until the present day. Early steps were taken by the Government and international agencies to buy and store seed for distribution and to finance grain deliveries to remote areas, but current water shortages have precipitated food, nutritional and health crises on an unprecedented scale, and primary care often consists largely of emergency measures. As the rains fail year after year, the variety of peoples who make up the Malian population have seen their livelihoods, animals and pastures gradually diminish. The nomadic Fulani and Tuareg groups have been forced to migrate and settle in the cities where they exist under marginal social and economic conditions typical of many peri-urban areas throughout the world. Previously concerned with animal husbandry, their lifestyles and social organization have had to change as they are forced to lead a sedentary and cultivating existence – neither of which have they had to do before. The result is that many of Mali's towns now have large 'floating populations' composed of a variety of ethnic groups with different social and economic structures and requirements.

Health expenditure is approximately 7.3% of the state budget, although much of this is focused on hospital-based western style health care systems in the urban areas, with three hospitals in Bamako (the capital) alone. In Mali, there was no decision to develop primary health care until late 1978. During the previous 15 years, however, basic primary care systems had been established from the grassroots upwards (in contrast to many countries who adopt a 'top-down' approach). In some areas, cooperatively funded village pharmacies were set up with the help of the national pharmaceutical organization, and their profits provided remuneration for the auxiliary midwives. Health posts were systematically constructed along with maternity units funded through regional tax levies. The community basis and support for the scheme, however, were lost in the regional centralization process. The rapid expansion seemed to occur at the expense of community involvement, and it appeared that 'even a regular drug supply is a burden on health resources and supply infrastructures' (McLean, 1984).

Social support services to back up medical care were also under-resourced. In late 1987, government 'fonctionnaires' (civil servants) in some towns had not been paid for many months, and morale and motivation to consolidate and extend services was very low. Transport and road networks are minimal, particularly during the rainy season, making access to small rural villages very difficult. The main problem, however, particularly in the north of the country in the fifth and sixth regions in the late part of 1987, was the continued failure of the rains and the destruction of the millet crop by drought leading to severe nutritional and food crises.

The following illustrates the services that are available:

Level (number)	Services	Health staff
Region (7)	Hospital (n=10, 3 of which are in Bamako)	
Cercle (46)	L'Assistance médicale de cercle	Doctor or nurse
Arrondissement (281)	Dispensaire rurale maternité	Nurse (curative) Nurse (preventive)
Villages (9482)	Centre de protection maternelle et infantile	

Staff shortages and maintaining trained staff in rural areas is a problem. In Bamako, the ratio of one doctor to every 25 000 people is exceeded in the rural areas where it is one doctor to every 115 000–390 000 people. Levels of community health development are low, partly because of a shortage of personnel, a lack of infrastructure including roads and communications networks and the inaccessibility of many groups, and partly because of the emergency nature of much of the care required. An 'équipe' of nurses and auxiliary workers tours the more accessible villages for about 20 days in the dry season (October–May) dealing with infectious diseases and vaccinations. In addition to this, teams of three part-time health workers are in the process of being trained – an auxiliary midwife, a village health worker and a health promoter (animatrice), the latter being concerned with prevention, health education and links with other sectors.

The importance of the *Expanded Programme of Immunization* has been recognized by the Malian Ministry of Health as being vital in reducing infant mortality rates. An evaluation by the Département d'Enseignement et Recherche en Santé Publique found that in some areas (the 'cercle' of Douentza in the fifth region for example) over 80% of the target population had been covered in the initial stages of the programme, especially for BCG, measles and the first dose of diphtheria and polio. The percentage of children receiving the second and third doses of diphtheria and polio is less, as a systematic call-up system is often difficult to instigate on a practical level. A survey conducted to find out reasons for non-vaccination found that the most frequently given reason was absence from the village rather than illness or a lack of awareness of the arrival of the mobile vaccination team. The lower figures for full vaccination for Douentza town (53%), compared with the surrounding rural areas (65.7%), could be accounted for by the fact that a very large percentage of Douentza's inhabitants consist of a 'floating population' – often Fulani or Tuareg groups who have moved down from the north with the encroaching drought and who move on again in search of work and opportunities – thus making the systematic organization of primary care more difficult to carry out. The rural villages in the 'cercle' are often composed of sedentary Fulani groups or Dogon people living in small communities along the escarpment and who tend to be less mobile or nomadic.

Another important aspect of primary care in the fifth region is the existence of the *Centres de Récuperation et d'Education Nutritionelle* (CRENs). These centres aim to provide a nutritious cooked porridge of maize flour, vegetable oil, powdered milk sugar and water to malnourished children (i.e. those under 80% weight for height). The mothers of the children in the CREN prepare the food and pay a small sum each month (about 20p) for transport, firewood etc. Local village health workers carry out the monitoring of weight for height, and treat sick children (aspirin, chloroquine and oral rehydration solution are all usually available).

Some problems encountered in the running of the CRENs include badly kept registers; no provision for destitute families whose children put on weight and are discharged only to be readmitted a few weeks later; children, whose state of health is related to illness rather than lack of food, are not always referred for proper treatment; the participation of the matronnes (health personnel) is unpaid and therefore has led to low motivation; the foodstuffs used in the CRENs are often either imported or not part of local diets – whereas the purchase of local food-stuffs would be more cost-effective.

Thus in Mali, the existence of integrated health care systems is somewhat sporadic due to the lack of general *infrastructure*, high rates of *mobility* of sections of the population, increasing *drought* and food shortages, and *varying motivation* of health personnel. As a result of the poorly integrated system of primary health care, health indices show high morbidity and mortality rates. Life expectancy is 43 years and infant mortality 175 per 1000 (1985). Proximity to the river delta has an effect on health for different groups. The Fulani who live in the delta all year round have higher child mortality rates than the Tuareg who move out in the rainy season. Infection rates are high and are suggested to contribute to the higher mortality for those remaining in the delta all year round (McLean, 1984; Hill, 1985).

Costa Rica

Costa Rica has a population of 2.7 million – of whom one half live in rural areas and one third are employed in agriculture. It has a history of progressive social developments over the last 100 years or so:

1869 – free mandatory primary education (now 92% literacy)

1880 – Jesuits expelled, religious communities prohibited, education became secular (now only 0.01% of the budget goes on the church)

1882 – elimination of the death penalty

1889 – beginnings of universal suffrage

1948 – free elections every four years, universal suffrage. During elections, a *Supreme Elections Tribunal* takes over power in the country with the police force under its authority. There is proportional representation and hence many small parties. If a party gets over 5% of the vote, the government pays their campaign funds at the next election.

1949 – abolition of the army; the police force is not a professional career

1978 – (and before) a policy of political asylum for people from, for example, Cuba, Chile, Nicaragua (10% of the population are refugees)

1983 – 50% of university students are women.

The country has a policy of political and ideological pluralism, social justice, and the solution of internal conflicts through dialogue and negotiation. There are vigorous social security, health and educational programmes, made possible by the abolition of the army – 27% of the budget is spent on education and culture. The terms 'disarmed democracy' and 'an island of peace in war-torn Central America' have been applied to Costa Rica.

The gross national product per head remains at about $1200 – it was reduced by the financial crisis of 1979–82 caused by a decrease in the prices of its main export products (coffee and bananas) and an increase in the price of oil, leading to short-term, high interest foreign loans.

Despite its financial difficulties, the health indices indicate that Costa Rica is achieving *developed* rather than *developing* country status – 78% of the population are covered by a social security system and 84% enjoy potable water services. Costa Rica has achieved phenomenal success in cutting its infant mortality rate from 84 per 1000 in 1960, 62 per 1000 in 1970 to 19 per 1000 in 1985. Comparisons with England and other Central American countries are given in Tables 10.2 and 10.3 below.

Table 10.2   *Comparisons with England (1984)*

	Costa Rica	England
Infant mortality rate (per 1000)	19	10
Life expectancy (years)	73	73
Per cent of babies born under 2500 g	6.5	6.9
Per cent of population aged 65+ years	3.7	15.0
Per cent of population aged under 15 years	36.2	6.3
Birth rate per 1000	33	12
Death rate per 1000	4	12
Health expenditure per person ($)	70	450

Source: DHSS (1986). *Health and Personal Social Services Statistics for England* London: HMSO Also: Jaramillo Antillón J. (1984). *Los Problemas de la Salud en Costa Rica.* San Jose: Min. de Salud.

Table 10.3   *Central American comparisons of infant mortality rates and child deaths at ages 1–4 years*

Age	Costa Rica	Death rates per 1000 (around 1980)				
		Guatemala	Honduras	Nicaragua	Panama	El Salvador
0–1 years	19	70	90	90	29	80
1–4 years	1	5	9	10	2	7

Source: Jaramillo Antillón J. (1984). *Los Problemas de la Salud en Costa Rica.* San Jose: Min. de Salud.

The large decrease in infant mortality rate since 1970 was due particularly to the introduction of improvements in primary health care. A sophisticated regression analysis of the factors involved in the infant mortality rate reduction from 1970 to 1980 showed that the following factors contributed in the proportions shown (Rosero-Bixby, 1985):

Socio-economic progress   22%
Fertility reduction   5%
Secondary care improvements   32%
Primary care improvements   41%

There is an additional dimension of health care of which Costa Rica is beginning to be aware – that is, with an increasing elderly population as a result of increasing life expectancy, the problems of chronic diseases of ageing and accidents begin to become important, as is the case in developed countries. At this stage, the treatment services rather than prevention play an increasing role, and there is the danger that the resources for them will be taken from those used for reducing morbidity and mortality.

In Costa Rica it was decided to adopt a pilot experiment using the key features of general practice as it is in the UK which are described in detail in Chapter 1. If there is anonymity and little continuity of care in the organization of the general practitioner service, patients and doctors can become dissatisfied. Self referral to hospital can lead to high hospitalization rates and duplication of treatment, while dissatisfaction of general practitioners can lead to high usage of investigations and medicines, all of which may result in high costs not only for general practice primary care services but also for the whole health service, leaving less resources available for preventive services.

PRIMARY HEALTH CARE PERSONNEL

Many primary health care programmes in all parts of the world utilize a variety of personnel in implementing and planning health strategies that are appropriate to local needs.

One of the most widespread workers is the *village health worker* who is chosen by the community as someone who is especially able and respected as a healer or leader. He or she may, for example, continue to work in the fields alongside the other village health workers but will spend about one hour a day providing health care. David Morley (1973) has suggested that training and support may be provided by the nearest health centre, and the health worker may be paid in part by the village community with one worker for every 500 people. If a health worker is appropriately selected, adequate support must be given at a national level to ensure the success of primary health care schemes. A nation's or government's commitment to primary health care can, in effect, be measured by the strength of this support which will determine the success or failure of the schemes.

The view of a part-time health worker accountable to his or her community in setting up a primary care network was reinforced by David Werner (1982) who established such a service in Mexico. He concluded that the village health worker:

(1) should be selected by the people from among themselves and should be responsible primarily to them and not to doctors and nurses.

(2) should be part-time and able therefore to subsist by performing agricultural or other work, possibly receiving a subsidy from the local community or national health service.

(3) may be somebody who has already been a traditional healer or birth attendant and should preferably be trained in the community – not only in curative but also in preventive and promotive functions.

In effect, the 'village health worker is a person from the community trained to function as a *bridge* between the community and the health care systems. The village health worker should be familiar with the health problems of the community and able to involve the people in identifying and confronting these problems, whilst improving their access to the government health service. From the outside, the village health worker can act as a facilitator for the arrival of appropriate medical intervention, health education and assistance in preventive care' (Liddell, 1985).

The village health worker may be wholly salaried, partly salaried, paid in kind or may work voluntarily; training varies in length and depth. In Niger, village health workers are given just ten days of practical training with a refresher course each year, whilst in Bangladesh training can last from one to 12 months. Tasks such as the following carried out by village health workers in Bangladesh are typical of most village health workers (Sanders, 1985):

(1) registration of births and deaths

(2) identification of pregnant women and identifying at-risk cases
(3) identification of at-risk children (e.g. children with malnutrition)
(4) immunization – BCG, diphtheria, pertussis, tetanus and polio
(5) nutrition and health education
(6) treatment of diarrhoea and dysentery; teaching and preparation of oral rehydration therapy
(7) motivation, supply and follow-up of family planning clients.

Thus, one of the main features of the village health worker's role is *preventive* work in addition to curative measures using low cost, easily available drugs or simple techniques, such as oral rehydration. Preventive measures may include malaria prophylaxis distribution or advice, identifying and monitoring those at risk from protein energy malnutrition (for example, by measuring upper arm circumference with a shakir strip) and providing nutritional supplement and rehabilitation. Broader preventive measures such as nutritional and agricultural monitoring, and the examination and improvement of clean water supplies, may also fall under the remit of the village health worker. It has been shown in many countries that the turnover of village health worker personnel is high, and that the transfer and retraining of personnel may have to be an integral part of a successful scheme.

In practice, the role of the village health worker is often carried out in conjunction with the *auxiliary*. Whereas the village health worker is selected by the community to augment basic health care knowledge through specific tasks and training, the task of the auxiliary is to extend the effectiveness of professional and paramedical care into the rural areas where most of the population live. Most categories of auxiliaries were developed to correspond to categories of professional and paramedical personnel – nursing, midwifery, environmental health and pharmaceutical – and thus have an important role to play in delivering primary care. Auxiliaries are usually wholly salaried, unlike the village health workers who often work voluntarily or receive payment in kind.

A number of problems have been evident in relation to the concept and practical role of the auxiliary. It has been shown that, after training, auxiliaries frequently do not remain in touch with the communities they intended to serve but often cater solely for 'important' people such as teachers and shop owners rather than the ordinary members of the community. The presence of auxiliaries has frequently not increased the use of local health services, and bureaucratic difficulties, such as in Mali, have often led to a high drop-out rate.

Many of the problems can perhaps be attributed to the fact that the auxiliary is first and foremost a *health professional* responsible in practice to the doctor above them in the professional hierarchy. The village health worker, however, is selected by the people of the community and as such is accountable and responsible to them. This is not to say that auxiliaries are always wholly inappropriate or operate unsuccessfully with the village health worker. The 'barefoot doctors' of China may serve as a model for the sort of medical auxiliaries needed in much of the developing world. There, selected members of every community are trained by mobile health teams, remaining in their own communities whilst gaining knowledge about simple medical treatment and general social and hygiene practices which are known to be causes of ill health.

MATERNAL AND CHILD HEALTH

One of the most important aspects of any primary health care strategy is the need for a coordinated and integrated programme of maternal and child health. In most developing countries, children and young adults under the age of 15 years make up about 40% of the population. If these were added to the number of expectant and lactating mothers then about 60% of the population would need to be covered by maternal and child health services (WHO, 1980).

In many ways, the aims of maternal and child health services are directly compatible with, if not the same as, the goals of overall community-based primary health care services but need to be specifically targeted to reach those sections of the population who may be low on the list of government priorities.

The general framework of maternal and child health principles is based on the notions that (Ebrahim, 1978):

(1) every expectant mother maintains good health, is prepared physically and psychologically to look after her child, goes through a normal delivery and bears a healthy child
(2) every child grows up in healthy surroundings, receives proper nourishment and adequate protection from disease
(3) communicable diseases are controlled in vulnerable groups by taking adequate preventive measures and by health education
(4) sickness is detected and treated early before it becomes serious or chronic

(5) simple statistical data on morbidity and mortality are maintained
at regional and national levels.

The role of *women* in many developing countries means that the
potential for both curative and preventive programmes focuses automatically on this group. 'Women are the vast untapped resource for
development' the World Health Organization declared in 1980. 'The
anchor for our strategies for health development should relate to all-
round improvement in the status of women and children who form the
majority of any population.' In addition, evidence has shown that the
health of mothers and their children is closely related to the health of
the community as a whole, and public health measures that will bring
about an improvement in general health will also provide maternal and
child health.

It is not only their maternal or child bearing role which makes
women effective targets for these programmes. Their overall responsibility for family health, their crucial economic status and social
influence are vital factors in maintaining and promoting basic primary
health care techniques. The United Nations *Decade for Women*
Conference in Nairobi in 1985 remarked that 'the eyes of health
planners began to turn towards women; as cooks; feeders of children;
as fetchers of water and firewood; as custodians of cleanliness and
hygiene; as teachers of healthy habits.' The conference disclosed that
'42 governments reported that they had expanded their maternal and
child health activities during the decade, with Senegal actually restruc-
turing its entire Ministry of Health to incorporate this new commitment.' Examples came from the Virgin Islands where pregnant women
and malnourished children are provided with margarine, wheat flour
and dried milk powder to supplement their diets, and in Guatemala
where one project giving supplementary food to pregnant women
reduced the incidence of low birth weight babies by 75%.

The importance of these simple but effective measures for reducing
infant mortality and overall morbidity rates must be set against a
background of general poor health indices for women, which start at
birth and continue throughout their lives. A United Nations study
found that, for selected rural areas in Africa, women in their last three
months of pregnancy actually lost weight − an average of 1.4 kg
each.

Furthermore, the state of women's health before they give birth is
seldom conducive to rapid recovery and fitness afterwards. Exhausting
work (African women carry out 60–80% of manual labour), multiple

pregnancies and nutritional shortfalls mean that overall health is unlikely to be good. In 1978, the World Health Organization found that 'two thirds of women in Asia, half of African women and one sixth of women in Latin America are anaemic', and that simple problems like this are often left untreated as 'two thirds of women in the developing world have no access to a trained health worker.'

This last point is illustrated by the fact that over half the world's births are attended by untrained traditional midwives or birth attendants who have acquired skills from their mothers, grandmothers and women in the community. In Sierra Leone, for example, 13 600 *traditional birth attendants* deliver 70% of the births, and 80% of births in Honduras are delivered by such women. Countries such as Honduras, however, have realized that additional primary health care training, building on the skills and social and cultural aspects of traditional birth attendants, provides a sound basis for establishing extensive antenatal and postnatal care. The United Nations Decade for Women Report estimated that India had provided additional training for a quarter of a million dais (traditional birth attendants) by 1981, Ethiopia had trained 47% of traditional midwives and Sri Lanka 95%. Benefits are reflected in mortality rates – in India, for example, deaths from neonatal tetanus were reduced dramatically in the three years following the dai training programme.

The special category of a *maternal and child health worker* is being phased out as it is recognized that the policies and premises of maternal and child health are best catered for within overall programmes of primary health care development. The World Health Organization (1980) has reported that a 'wide range of workers from various sectors both formal and informal are being considered for maternal and child health care. At the community level these would include primary health care workers, crèche staff, extension workers, members of women's organizations and traditional birth attendants.'

FAMILY PLANNING

The issue of family planning in the developing world is often a contentious one, frequently because it is seen by developed countries as a panacea for more profound social, economic and resource problems in the Third World, or because programmes may have been carried out insensitively or without adequate information, especially for women.

Family planning does, however, have a very important part to play in reducing maternal mortality rates and improving the health of children – and indeed, in counteracting unrestrained population growth. The World Health Organization recently showed that 'in developing countries today about 5.6 million infant deaths and 200 000 maternal deaths could be avoided if women chose to have their children within the safest years with adequate spacing and completed families of moderate size' (Archer, 1985).

Not only is maternal mortality associated with pregnancies in very young women, but repeated child bearing takes its toll through anaemia, malnutrition and infection. Furthermore, children born following high risk pregnancies, particularly when they occur less than two years apart, are likely to have a low birth weight, to die in infancy or to suffer from infection or malnutrition in childhood.

It is estimated that some 360 million women world-wide do not use any form of contraception and, as a result, have larger numbers of children than they would prefer. The *Nepal Contraceptive Prevalence Survey* of 1981 found that the mean actual family size was 5.9, although the mean desired family size was 4.4. In Sri Lanka, it was found that the mean actual family size was 5.0 whilst the mean desired family size was 3.2 (Archer, 1985).

Several major difficulties exist with regard to the implementation of family planning methods in developing countries. Firstly, in the absence of widespread systems of social security, residential or respite care for the elderly and the high economic importance of children as labour and inheritors, family planning and limiting of numbers of children may be seen as jeopardizing the security of the family as a whole. Secondly, *religious* or *cultural* reasons and pressure from men may deter women from taking up facilities. In Mexico, for example, the Roman Catholic church announced that every person who undergoes sterilization will be excommunicated.

The variety of methods available also poses problems for many women. One of the most controversial is the widespread use of *injectable contraceptives* in the developing world. Depo-medroxypro-gesterone acetate marketed as Depo-Provera by Upjohn, and norethis-terone enanthate marketed as Norigest (or norethisterone oenanthate marketed as Noristerate) by Schering, have caused much controversy. Although they are simple to use and their use can be kept secret (an important consideration for many women), injectables may cause significant menstrual disturbances in many users and amenorrhoea may persist for weeks after the last dose. *Oral contraceptives* have also caused some controversy as to their side-effects, and although they have low method failure, they may have high user failure as many women find it difficult to regulate their lives to the degree necessary to remember to take the pill each day.

Intra-uterine devices (IUDs) may also be problematic in that specialized training is necessary for their insertion, infection rates are high and in Islamic countries, for example, vaginal examination particularly by a man is prohibited. In Bali, a predominantly Hindu island where it is not unusual to have male traditional birth attendants, there is little objection to using IUDs on religious or cultural grounds. In contrast, the neighbouring island of Java is strongly Muslim, and of the new family planning acceptors, only one fifth as many choose IUDs as choose oral contraceptives or injectables.

POLITICAL, PLANNING AND FINANCIAL CONSIDERATIONS

One of the main features of successful primary health care services is its *cost-effectiveness*. This is generally assessed by examining whether the needs of the majority of the population are being met in the most efficient way. This may, as already discussed, involve a degree of change in terms of political commitment to focus on groups who may be politically powerless, economically underprivileged or socially marginalized. Political disputes may take place at a local as well as a national level. Furthermore, the urban elite and politically powerful may support in theory the extension of primary health care services to rural areas as long as the city facilities remain unchanged. Since these services swallow up a disproportionately large amount of the health budget, this is often impossible and serves to emphasize the need to transfer some resources from overprivileged urban areas and into rural communities.

Overall budgeting for health is often not a top priority for many governments and indeed, the formation of a 'national health policy' may be a new concept for many political leaders. Furthermore, the health ministry has to compete with other ministries for resources and will usually have a lower status than defence or foreign affairs. In

Honduras in 1985, spending on health and education fell to less than 7% of the national budget whilst military spending consumed 30%. Cost-effectiveness must take into consideration *capital* and *recurrent costs*. The former may comprise the construction of hospitals, health centres and pharmacy buildings together with, perhaps, roads to reach them, electricity and water supplies, which in themselves incur running costs. Wages for health personnel, training and skill development can prove expensive in the long-term. Moreover, the balance between the local and national orientation of services must consider the phenomenon of increasing demand with increasing availability. As with many other commodities, 'in many developing countries the demand may be relatively low because there is not much health care available. One can expect that by increasing the supply of health care new demand will be created' (Zschock, 1979).

Drugs and their selection are also of importance. The selection of a limited number in relation to epidemiological patterns and control of prevalent diseases must be of paramount importance. In many countries, a severe shortage of cheap, effective and easily administered drugs is often coupled with oversupply of expensive preparations which can often do more harm than good. In Honduras, one auxiliary reported 'two cases of children who were critically ill as the result of being given the wrong medication. One had been given sulphadiazine and developed renal complications and another had been given dipyrone for a fever. The drugs were bought in large pharmacies in Santa Barbara as individual tablets without indications for use by people who largely cannot read anyway' (Liddell, 1985).

Effective primary health care development involves a large element of *decentralization* of both planning and decision making. It has been remarked that 'district level involvement in planning can help close the gap between the plan and the reality'. Local health personnel interacting with officials from other organizations (agricultural or community organizations, for example) will often be better placed to find workable responses to local problems than higher placed officials in the national capital. An evaluation by the US Agency for International Development (USAID) found that 'training workers as physician extenders represents for most countries a major change in service delivery. Some countries, such as Tunisia or Lesotho, have had to enact special legislation to authorize non-physicians to provide health care' (USAID, 1984).

Planning must also seek to strike a balance between *curative* and *preventive* care. Walt and Vaughan (1981) have remarked that 'people want to be treated and cured not told what to do to prevent illness, or worse what should have been done to prevent their illness. A good health worker may be inundated with patients, leaving no time for preventive work where the results are slower and harder to appreciate. At higher levels, there are always conflicting demands in the allocation of resources, on acute versus chronic care and on cure versus prevention.'

A study of 50 USAID assisted projects world-wide in 1984, concluded that often 'communities feel no strong need for the primary health care programmes that are being offered because their curative needs are already being met through established channels, and they do not place a high priority on the preventive services which the programmes seek to introduce.'

SOCIAL AND CULTURAL FACTORS

Establishing and operating a primary health care system often highlights the need for substantial social and economic change and reorganization at a variety of levels. An important factor in all developing countries is that the widespread existence of malnutrition is not directly attributable to ignorance or mismanagement of diet but more directly to *poverty* and lack of purchasing power. 'Poverty means that people cannot afford enough food – it also puts people in an unhygienic environment. Living in a slum shelter or in a one-roomed house in a village makes it impossible to prepare food cleanly and to avoid infection and the transmission of parasites' (Wheeler and Khanum, 1985).

Thus, primary health care at a village level necessitates collaboration with a variety of other national and local government departments, not only to prevent but also to *predict* health and nutritional crises. For example in Dacca, Bangladesh, Save the Children Fund workers found that 'a health centre responsible for a defined population would need to work closely with the agricultural services in identifying nutritional problems and in finding appropriate solutions, or in analysing seasonal interrelationships between agricultural and labour demands and disease incidence and supply and distribution problems, or in mitigating or controlling occupational health hazards from resettlement programmes or irrigation schemes' (Wheeler and Khanum, 1985).

By assessing these criteria, responses to health crises can potentially be decided in advance. In many Sahel countries, for example, a rise or fluctuation in market prices, the selling of possessions or livestock, or migrations of groups of people are now monitored to prevent famine disasters such as that which occurred on a massive scale in 1984. Improving the political and economic power of the landless poor may improve their health in Bangladesh, whilst in Mali a lack of roads and transport services hampers community-based development.

Raising overall *educational standards* and levels of literacy are vital for improving knowledge about self-care and preventive techniques. Throughout the world, 82% of boys and 71% of girls of primary school age are in school – an increase of 7% and 11%, respectively, since 1975. It has been found, for example, that 'women with more than seven years of education are four times as likely to use contraception in countries as different as Kenya, Bangladesh and Mexico.' As the use of contraception goes up, so the birth rate goes down, and this in turn increases the chances of individual children receiving the kind of care they need. In fact, the United Nations Decade for Women Conference remarked that 'women's ability to read and write has been discovered to be a better way of predicting their children's health than even their income.'

Initiating and augmenting such profound social changes are not always a priority for many governments who may challenge the assertiveness and self-reliance of many communities if they are seen to be threatening the centralized influence of the politically powerful elite. Primary health care as a concept must also be seen to identify and reinforce positive elements of *indigenous* systems of health care, and to adapt to and incorporate the spiritual and religious concepts of health and illness in various societies whilst raising awareness of potentially harmful practices. In Honduras, for example ' "ojo" (evil eye) is a condition of small infants that may be characterized by fever or diarrhoea. An infant suffers "ojo" if stared at by a "strong" person such as a sweating man or a pregnant woman. Prevention is achieved by wearing red clothes or a charm' (Liddell, 1985). Similarly, West African 'marabouts' may cure illnesses 'caused' by grudges or bad feeling with the use of 'gri-gri' (charms) or by referring the patient to specific sections of the Koran. These cultural and spiritual beliefs and values must be taken into account sensitively by planners and primary health care workers. The instantaneous inclusion of western values and attitudes to health as part of a primary health care 'package' amounts to no more than an inappropriate, patronizing approach and does little to encourage effective and appropriate development.

GLOBAL PERSPECTIVE

A discussion of the development and appropriateness of primary health care in the developing world must be placed in the overall context of international global development. The filtering down of primary health care services to a community level can really be initiated only by national government commitment and, perhaps, inter-governmental collaboration.

Why some countries stay poor, and why certain groups in certain countries stay very poor, is bound up with the question not only of internal power distribution but also of *international financial co-operation and debt*. 'The Third World is facing an unprecedented financial crisis with its debt growing exponentially whilst its export earnings are plummeting . . . such a crisis was by no means accidental given the mathematical imperatives of borrowing and the role played in global lending by the transnational circuit. Simply put, the more that is borrowed, the more that needs to be borrowed' (Cavanagh, 1986). As the development of primary health care systems cannot take place outside the overall economic and financial infrastructure of developing countries, priorities are not likely to be given to new, untried, innovative schemes which may act as catalysts for social change on a higher level if the existing political organization is itself under threat from international financial pressures.

Of the three major regions, Latin America dominates the debt scene with US$368 billion (46%), Asia US$304 billion and Africa US$129 billion. Whilst total African debt is only 16% of the total debt service of most African economies, it is huge in relation to each of the countries' gross domestic product. In 1984, President Julius Nyerere of Tanzania remarked at the Commonwealth Conference 'Africa's debt burden is now intolerable. We cannot pay. You know it and all our creditors know it. It is not a rhetorical question when I ask should we really let out people starve so we can pay our debts.' The size of these debts has thus limited many countries' options for development and increased their dependence on external aid, curtailing the number and nature of long-term health care projects designed to minimize present and future health crises. National budgets may be so deeply steeped in debt repayments that health may be way down the list of priorities – after, for example, military expenditure. International hostilities and offensives may also jeopardize primary care development at a local level – in Mozambique for example, it has been suggested that South African government-backed rebel offensives disrupt local health care facilities and famine relief operations.

Other international *political* and *economic* considerations can also have an effect on the nature of primary care development at a local level. 'Agribusiness', or the role of multinational corporations which deal in the production and distribution of foodstuffs, can also have a direct effect on health by, for example, causing the substitution of subsistence crops by cash crops for export, which may lead not only to social and economic reorganization but also to ecological and environmental changes and thus affect nutritional and health indicators.

Primary health care cannot, therefore, be considered outside the global political and economic influences on development and change. International collaboration has the power to advise, motivate and innovate but it also has the power to weaken, destabilize and destroy modes of economic and social organization in the developing world that are closely linked with health and health care.

THE FUTURE

It has been established that primary health care can build on individual and collective responsibility for health by both informing and motivating populations. Where successful primary health care development goes hand in hand with other aspects of social and economic change on a broader level, such as in Costa Rica, the results can be very effective. In many countries, however, primary health care is often a luxury or at least a purchasable commodity used as a political football in intra- and inter-governmental conflict. Primary health care thus implies a commitment to a political goal which may see much opposition and a shift of emphasis of government policy, but is in itself a *system* by which services may be delivered regularly and reliably to the majority of the population at an affordable cost.

If primary health care is successfully established, and overall improvements in the geneal health of the population are achieved, repercussions up through the hierarchy of health services will ensue. The more efficient use of hospital services may mean that fewer specialists are required; preventive health care will need a continual supply of educational and informative material; the ageing, and particularly the elderly, population will require health systems appropriate to their needs – possibly more like UK general practice; the expanding group of young people will need increased educational and employment opportunities; and there will be the need for a safety net of a social security system for those who are unable to cope economically. Increased western influences on many nations bring with them an increase in – for example – smoking, and epidemiological patterns may show 'western' trends with increased lung cancer or heart disease.

REFERENCES AND FURTHER READING

Archer E. (1985). *Injectable Contraceptives*. London: The Save the Children Fund.

Cavanagh J. (1987). Impossible debt on the road to global ruin. *The Guardian*, 9 Jan, 1987.

Chen L. C. (1986). Primary health care in developing countries – overcoming operational and social barriers. *Lancet*, II, 1260–5.

Ebrahim G. J. (1978). *Practical Mother and Child Health in Developing Countries*. London: Macmillan.

Ebrahim G. J. (1985). *Social and Community Paediatrics in Developing Countries*. London: Macmillan.

Halstead S. B., Walsh J. A., Warren J. A., eds. (1985). *Good Health at Low Cost*. New York: Rockefeller Foundation.

Joseph S. C. (1985). The case for clinical services. In *Good Health at Low Cost* (Halstead S. B., Walsh J. A., Warren J. A. eds.) pp. 221–7. New York: Rockefeller Foundation.

Liddell W. G. (1985). *The Study of Village Health Workers in Santa Barbara, Honduras*. London: The Save the Children Fund.

McLean W. (1984). *Mali – Country Profile*. Working paper – Food Emergencies Research Unit, Department of Human Nutrition, London School of Hygiene and Tropical Medicine.

Morley D. (1973). *Paediatric Priorities in the Developing World*. London: Butterworths.

Rosero-Bixby L. (1985). Infant mortality decline in Costa Rica in Halstead et al (1985).

Sanders D. (1986). *The Struggle for Health, Medicine and the Politics of Underdevelopment*. London: Macmillan.

United Nations (1985). *The State of the World's Women 1985.* Report of the *UN Decade for Women Conference,* Nairobi 1985. Oxford: New Internationalist Publications.

United Nations International Children's Emergency Fund – UNICEF (1987). *The State of the World's Children 1986.* Oxford: New Internationalist Publications.

United States Agency for International Development (1984). *An Evaluation of 50 USAID Assisted Projects.* Washington DC: USAID.

Walt G., Vaughan P. (1981). *An Introduction to Primary Health Care in Developing Countries.* London: London School of Hygiene and Tropical Medicine.

Werner D., Bower B. (1982). *Helping Health Workers Learn.* Palo Alto, California: Hesperian Foundation.

Wheeler E., Khanum S. (1985). *Nutrition and Malnutrition in Bangladesh.* Children's Nutritional Unit (CNU) Training Manual. London: The Save the Children Fund.

World Health Organization (1978). *Declaration of Alma-Ata.* Report of the *International Conference on Primary Health Care,* Alma-Ata, USSR, 1978. Geneva: WHO.

World Health Organization (1980). *Towards a Better Future; Maternal and Child Health.* Geneva: WHO.

Zschock D. K. (1979). *Health Care Financing in Developing Countries.* Washington DC: American Public Health Association International Health Programme.

Index